I0559522

# Sensual Symphony

## EMBRACING FEMININE SENSUALITY

# HANNA OLIVAS

ALONG WITH 6 INSPIRING WOMEN AUTHORS

© **2024 ALL RIGHTS RESERVED**.

Published by She Rises Studios Publishing **www.SheRisesStudios.com.**

No part of this book may be reproduced or transmitted in any form whatsoever, electronic, or mechanical, including photocopying, recording, or by any informational storage or retrieval system without the expressed written, dated and signed permission from the publisher and co-authors.

LIMITS OF LIABILITY/DISCLAIMER OF WARRANTY:

The co-authors and publisher of this book have used their best efforts in preparing this material. While every attempt has been made to verify the information provided in this book, neither the co-authors nor the publisher assumes any responsibility for any errors, omissions, or inaccuracies.

The co-authors and publisher make no representation or warranties with respect to the accuracy, applicability, or completeness of the contents of this book. They disclaim any warranties (expressed or implied), merchantability, or for any purpose. The co-authors and publisher shall in no event be held liable for any loss or other damages, including but not limited to special, incidental, consequential, or other damages.

ISBN: 978-1-964619-36-1

# TABLE OF CONTENTS

# INTRODUCTION

Welcome to *Sensual Symphony: Embracing Feminine Sensuality*. As you open these pages, you are stepping into a world where sensuality is celebrated not as a mere physical trait but as a rich, harmonious blend of your entire being—physical, emotional, and spiritual. This book is an invitation to reconnect with and embrace the multifaceted essence of your femininity, allowing it to illuminate your life in profound and empowering ways.

In our fast-paced, often dissonant world, the true symphony of our sensuality can become drowned out by external pressures and internal doubts. Yet, within each of us lies a powerful, beautiful rhythm that connects us to our deepest selves and to those around us. This book aims to help you rediscover and honor that rhythm, and to embrace sensuality as a natural, vital part of who you are.

You will find within these pages a blend of insightful reflections and practical exercises designed to guide you on a journey of self-love and body positivity. We will explore topics such as intimacy, pleasure, and the art of seduction—each framed within the broader context of celebrating the feminine essence. Through engaging anecdotes and thoughtful guidance, *Sensual Symphony* seeks to inspire a renewed appreciation for your sensual self, encouraging you to integrate this awareness into every facet of your life.

This journey is not just about enhancing personal pleasure but also about enriching your relationships, sparking creativity, and fostering a deeper sense of well-being. By embracing your sensuality, you open the door to a more vibrant and fulfilling existence.

As you embark on this exploration, remember that sensuality is not a destination but a continuous, evolving experience. It is about celebrating the beauty of your body, the depth of your desires, and the power of your pleasures. Let this book be your guide to a more connected, empowered, and joyous self. Welcome to your Sensual Symphony.

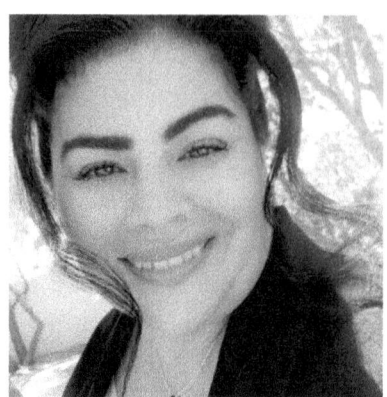

## Hanna Olivas

Founder and CEO of She Rises Studios

https://www.linkedin.com/company/she-rises-studios/
https://www.facebook.com/sherisesstudios
https://www.instagram.com/sherisesstudios_llc/
www.SheRisesStudios.com

Author, Speaker, and Founder. Hanna was born and raised in Las Vegas, Nevada, and has paved her way to becoming one of the most influential women of 2022. Hanna is the co-founder of She Rises Studios and the founder of the Brave & Beautiful Blood Cancer Foundation. Her journey started in 2017 when she was first diagnosed with Multiple Myeloma, an incurable blood cancer. Now more than ever, her focus is to empower other women to become leaders because The Future is Female. She is currently traveling and speaking publicly to women to educate them on entrepreneurship, leadership, and owning the female power within.

# Sensuality as a Symphony: A Journey of Harmony, Power, and Feminine Grace

By Hanna Olivas

There are moments in life that take us by surprise, moments that invite us to lean in, listen, and truly feel. For me, sensuality has always been more than a surface-level experience—it is a symphony. Each note, each movement, and each breath is part of a melody that has carried me through the seasons of my life. It's a rhythm that flows deep within me, guiding how I engage with the world, myself, and those I love. Sensuality isn't just about physical touch; it is the vibration of life itself. It is an orchestral performance of the mind, body, and spirit working together, playing the most intimate music that only I can hear. But when it is heard, truly heard by another—something magical happens. When I think of sensuality, I don't think of it as something external. It isn't about how we dress, how we move, or the things we say to invoke desire. Sensuality, for me, is an internal energy, one that pulses from my very core. It's the way I experience life through every sense: the way my skin feels against the breeze, the taste of something sweet and forbidden on my lips, the scent of jasmine in the night air, and the sight of beauty in unexpected places. Every touch, taste, sight, smell, and sound contributes to the score that makes up my life. Growing up, I didn't always understand sensuality this way. I was raised in an environment where sensuality wasn't openly discussed, and yet, it lived in the quiet spaces between the words that weren't spoken. I learned to observe, listen, and discover that the things left unsaid could carry a deeper meaning than what was spoken aloud. I found myself drawn to the subtleties of life, to the way the world could feel so alive and electric in the simplest of moments. But it wasn't until later in life that I fully understood how to access my own sensuality, how to use it not just as a way to connect with others, but as a way to connect with myself. Sensuality is the symphony that plays within us all, and like any symphony, it requires time to learn and practice. At first, I stumbled through it, not always knowing how to express it, sometimes too afraid to embrace it. There were times I felt I didn't deserve to feel such pleasure in life, that there were other things more important than indulging in the luxuries of the senses. But then, there came a moment—a moment that changed everything. It was a night like any other, but it also felt like the beginning of something. The air was thick with anticipation, though I didn't yet know what it was I was waiting for. As I walked outside, the moonlight wrapped around me like a soft silk robe, and the world seemed to pause. I remember the feeling of the cool grass beneath my bare feet, the scent of night-blooming flowers carried by the breeze, and the way the stars above seemed to pulse in time with my heartbeat. Everything was quiet, and yet everything felt alive, vibrating with possibility. In that moment, I realized that sensuality isn't something that happens to us—it's something we create. It's the symphony we compose with each breath we take, each step we make, and each moment we allow ourselves to be fully present in our bodies. Sensuality is about owning the space we occupy, feeling the energy around us, and using that energy to fuel our desires, our dreams, and our passions. It's about moving through the world with intention, with grace, and with a deep sense of knowing that we are deserving of every pleasure life has to offer. I began to understand that sensuality is power. It is the power to be fully in control of my own body, my own mind, and my own desires. It is the power to say yes to the things that excite me and no to the things that do not serve me. It is the power to take up space, to be seen, to be heard, and to be felt. Sensuality is a dance with life—a dance that requires both surrender and strength. It's about giving in to the flow, allowing yourself to be carried by the rhythm, while also knowing when to take the lead. As I continued to explore my own sensuality, I discovered that it is deeply intertwined with creativity. The more I allowed myself to indulge in the pleasures of life, the more creative I became. Writing, for me, is a deeply sensual act. It is a way for me to express the things I feel but cannot always say aloud. The words flow from me like music, each one carrying a note of emotion, of passion, of desire. Writing allows me to tap into that deep well of sensuality within me and share it with the world. It is a way for me to connect with others on a level that goes beyond the surface, a way for me to invite others into my world, to feel what I feel, and to experience what I experience. Sensuality is also about connection—not just with ourselves but with others. It's about the way we touch, the way we speak, the way we look into someone's eyes and let them see us for who we truly are. It's about the way we allow ourselves to be vulnerable, to be open, to be seen. And when we do that, when we allow ourselves to be fully present in our bodies, our emotions, and our desires, something magical happens. We create a space for intimacy, connection, and love. There is something profoundly erotic about being fully in tune with yourself, about knowing what you want and allowing yourself to take it. Sensuality is about pleasure, yes, but it's also about joy. It's about finding joy in the simplest of things—the feel of a soft blanket against your skin, the taste of chocolate melting on your tongue, the sound of rain tapping against the window. These small moments of pleasure, when added together, create a symphony of joy that fills every corner of your life. For me, sensuality is a celebration of the feminine. It is a way to honor the body, the mind, and the spirit. It is about embracing the curves of my body, the softness of my skin, and the depth of my emotions. It is about recognizing the power that comes from being a woman, from being connected to the cycles of the moon, the earth, and the universe. Sensuality is a reminder that we are not separate from the world around us—we are part of it. We are connected to the earth, to the stars, and to each other. And it is through this connection that we find our power. In my journey, I've learned that sensuality isn't something to be ashamed of—it's something to be celebrated. It is a gift, one that allows us to experience the world in a way that is rich, full, and vibrant. It is a way for us to reclaim our power, our joy, and our pleasure. And when we do that, when we fully embrace our sensuality, we become unstoppable. As women, we are often told to tone it down, to hide our desires, to be modest. But I say, why? Why should we dim our light? Why should we deny ourselves the pleasure that life has to offer? We deserve to feel joy, to feel pleasure, to feel alive. We deserve to be the conductors of our own symphonies, to create a life that is full of beauty, passion, and love. So, my dear sisters, I invite you to join me on this journey of sensuality. I invite you to step into your power, to embrace your desires, and to allow yourself to feel everything. I invite you to create your own symphony, one that is uniquely yours, one that reflects the beauty, the strength, and the grace that lives within you. Sensuality is not something to be feared—it is something to be celebrated. It is a reminder that we are alive, that we are powerful, and that we deserve every pleasure life has to offer. Let the music of your sensuality play. Let it fill every corner of your life. Let it guide you, inspire you, and empower you. For you are a symphony, my love, and the world is waiting to hear your song.

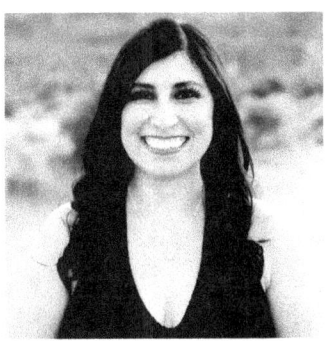

## Ana Martinez

A New Adventure
Peer to Peer Mentor

https://www.linkedin.com/in/anamlv
https://www.facebook.com/anarnclc
https://www.instagram.com/anam.rnclc/
https://www.anewadventurelv.com/
https://calendly.com/anamlv/30min

Ana is a mom of three beautiful daughters, Registered Nurse, Certified Lactation Counselor, Travel Specialist, and How Money Works Educator. She is an Honors College graduate from the University of Nevada Las Vegas in 2013 with a Bachelor of Science in Nursing. She devoted a decade to nursing across various specialties, including labor, delivery, postpartum, and hospice care. She became a Certified Lactation Counselor in 2017 and driven by her passion for travel, she became a Travel Specialist in 2022. In 2024, she transitioned to entrepreneurship in the financial industry alongside the travel and wellness industries. Her mission is to empower her community with their prenatal, travel, and financial well-being.

In her free time, she enjoys dancing and traveling, enriching her life with diverse experiences and creative pursuits.

Life is too short to settle for anything less than extraordinary, especially when it comes to living authentically as your true self.

# Living a Sensual Life

By Ana Martinez

## Female Sensuality

As women, were we taught to understand our female sensuality when we were girls? I know I was not. I believe my mom and grandma did not know what our female sensuality was or entailed and confused it with sexuality as prior generations of women before them. According to a quick Google search, sensuality is the enjoyment, expression, or pursuit of physical, especially sexual, pleasure or the condition of being pleasing or fulfilling to the senses. Like Google, many people, including my family, associate sensuality with sexuality when it should be associated with the senses, our human senses of taste, hearing, sight, smell, and touch. Thus, growing up my mom focused on academics, ingraining the expectation of obtaining higher education and physical puberty changes like body odor or the fact that I would get a period. But, there was no talk about feminine energy vs masculine energy, becoming a high-value woman, or the hormone changes that would initiate feelings of sexual desire.

## Feminine vs. Masculine Energy

Feminine energy is a spiritual force that is said to be connected to positive traits like compassion, empathy, and introspection according to Google. Feminine energy is passive energy, the state of being, going with the flow, receiving rather than doing, attracting rather than chasing. It is the opposite of masculine energy, which is expressed when someone is working toward a goal, making progress, or pushing forward. Feminine energy is expressed when someone moves with the flow of life, lets situations be, uses the law of least effort, embraces creative energy, and tunes into their internal process. Typically, a woman would have feminine energy with a dab of masculine energy as demonstrated by a routine which acts like the guards in a bowling lane so we may flow within those parameters. While men would typically have masculine energy with a dab of feminine energy to have empathy for others.

## High-Value Woman

Growing up I was taught by my mom that a high-value woman was a woman who had a good reputation, was independent, had a great job, and did not need a man. I was taught there was one way to live and that was to seek higher education and gain a degree that would be reliable. Yet, according to Google it is someone who has high self-esteem; knows her worth, stands up for herself, has very high emotional intelligence, embraces her femininity, and is self-confident. That is a significant difference between what I was led to believe and what I am now learning to strive for.

After the birth of my third baby, subsequent postpartum depression and anxiety, therapy, couples therapy, moving to Oklahoma for one month with the in-laws, and many ups and downs with my partner, I was able to find the education I needed to grow as a human being into a high-value woman who understands her female sensuality and energy. I give credit to my partner, Maternal Minds Counseling, Lisa Glamour and Vickita Trivedi on YouTube who helped with my development. My goal is to share what I have learned by sharing my story and four steps to guide you through your journey to understand your sensuality and feminine energy, and become a high-value woman.

## My Story

## High School

In high school, I had my first long-term boyfriend. As a 15-year-old girl, I was fascinated by his physique. He was athletic and had a six-pack. We both ran cross country and had plans to seek higher education. He was my first sexual partner and we enjoyed being intimate. It was so out of control that my mom caught us at least twice. However, I was responsible enough to let my mom know when I began being sexually active to get on birth control. We went to Planned Parenthood and I was given Plan B and a Depo injection. I remained on Depo for many years and avoided getting pregnant.

## University

I quickly met my former husband in the nursing program weeks after breaking up with my high school boyfriend. Moving forward, we graduated from nursing school and he wanted to get married to avoid living in sin as he was a devout Roman Catholic. I was born and raised Roman Catholic, but I was more of an Easter and Christmas Catholic. Thus, to get married in the Catholic church, I had to undergo the sacrament of confession and stop birth control as it is considered a mortal sin. One month after our wedding, I was pregnant. My mom was disappointed as she expected me to continue higher education. However, my former husband and I took the initiative to get educated. We decided to have an intervention-free birth and ended up hiring a Certified Professional Midwife to have a homebirth.

## Homebirth

For the first time, I felt empowered. I trained my body and mind and manifested the birth I wanted with the help of the Bradley Method. Yes, it was painful. Yet, I was surrounded by women who held space for me to labor and birth my baby the way I wanted to bring her into this world. I was so scared I would not love my baby because I never grew up wanting to be a mother. In fact, growing up my mom never encouraged motherhood as a plan. It was always about academics. Thus, I needed as much oxytocin, the love hormone, to bond with my baby.

When she was born, I remember her coming out and the midwife positioning her into my arms. I was so tired and I was disappointed in myself for not feeling a sense of love at first sight as many other women promised me I would feel. I felt guilty. It took me a couple of days to feel love. Breastfeeding helped me despite the lack of support from my family. Fast-forward and it was a tough postpartum. It was full of postpartum depression and anxiety. My marriage crumbled despite couples therapy and trying different antidepressants. Both of us were under so much stress and after much struggle, we decided to separate.

## Mom's Death

A month and a half later, my mom fell seriously ill. Come to find out she had colon cancer. The tumor burst. After eight days of hospitalization, surgery, many interventions, and hospice for her last 24 hours, my mom died in the middle of my divorce. I did not have time to grieve. I had a two-year-old to take care of, navigate co-parenting, and figure out my mom's mortuary arrangements along with sorting out any pending business she had left. That was one of the most challenging times in my life. I was alone. My mom was my best friend. I had never regretted being an only child until my mom died. On the days I did not have my daughter, I went out. I ended up meeting my current partner during that time and became friends with benefits. As months went by we became friends. I got pregnant, he moved in, and I had my second homebirth. When my second daughter turned one, I got pregnant for the third and last time. I had so much postpartum depression and anxiety from the current stressors, lack of support, and the unknown that I decided it was for the best to obtain a tubal ligation. I was blessed to have a gynecologist who performed the procedure and had no complications. Afterwards, I felt a sense of freedom. I did not have to worry about getting pregnant anymore.

# How Does My Story Fit into Female Sensuality?

Many women do not receive the education necessary to understand their sensuality; thus, making mistakes along the way. As shown in my story, I lived in masculine energy for so, so long. I took on roles I did not need to take. Analyzing my behavior, I was expressing my sensuality via sexuality. I had no compass or role model to express my sensuality in other ways. My younger self was afraid to be alone. I lacked self-awareness and self-love to make decisions that would make ME happy. I did not have the confidence to focus on myself, learn who I was outside of a romantic relationship, and become a high-value, feminine woman. It was easier to follow others' decisions than voice my opinion. After so many years of looking at the past with regret, I am continuously learning to enjoy my present and learn and heal from my past.

Here are four steps that will be broken down and explained to help guide you through your journey to understand your sensuality and feminine energy, and become a high-value woman.

## Step 1: The Mind

### Mindset and Mental Discipline

We need to work on changing our mindset and practicing mental discipline. What does that mean? In a nutshell, no negative self-talk. In the beginning, it will take a lot of mental discipline to stop ourselves from having a negative, close-minded perspective. We are in a constant battle with ourselves, the ego vs our higher self. The ego, according to Google, is a person's sense of self-esteem or self-importance. It is the part of the mind that mediates between the conscious mind and the unconscious and is responsible for reality testing and a sense of personal identity. It is the sense of our own worth. Next, we have our higher self. That part of ourselves that is seeking opportunity, that believes in ourselves, and pushes us to uncomfortable places. The ego is louder and keeps us safe, but if we listen to it, we will not grow to our full potential. The ego is fed by giving it our attention; thus, we need to start ignoring it. But, how? By letting go of negative beliefs, embracing a positive self-concept/image of yourself, social media, healing from past trauma, gaining financial independence, using your imagination, and learning the maybe; this or better philosophy. In a nutshell, ask, "What is easier? What path will bring less active energy?" Remember that being a woman is enough, we are the source of life. Living in peace and letting things be is a mindset to strive for.

## Letting Go of Negative Beliefs and Embracing a Positive Self-Concept/Image

As we grow up, we have negative beliefs that either we came up with ourselves or that we were told by others. If it is a negative belief, we need to start reframing those beliefs that are not serving us and let them go (which is easier said than done). How do we do that? We need to begin by acknowledging that negative belief and voice it out loud. If we keep ignoring those beliefs, we cannot fix them, reframe them, and let them go. Our minds and thus beliefs which become thoughts and words are so powerful and want to prove us right. For example, when you believe or say "I am ugly" your mind will find ways to prove to you that you are ugly. Your mind will uphold that image and your actions and habits will lead to you wearing clothes that make you look ugly or become lazy to maintain yourself with unhealthy habits to prove you right. Thus, the need to work on letting go of the negative beliefs, thoughts, and words and embrace a positive self-concept/image. A great way to handle negative beliefs and thoughts is to write them down. Voicing out loud our beliefs or thoughts is good, but writing them down is even better. It is like siphoning out the poison from our minds. As a mother, I have dealt with many self-doubts about my parenting style and/or when overwhelmed or overstimulated, wanting to run away from my responsibilities. Journaling has helped me write out my doubts and clear my mind as to what I really want, which is to be the best mom I can be to my daughters.

As time goes on, it will take less mental discipline to one, acknowledge and notice your thoughts and words, and two, if negative, stop the negativity. It will become more habitual and like when flipping TV channels, be able to flip to positive thoughts or words in an instant. During those times when you notice yourself having negative thoughts or words of yourself, here are some self-care affirmations from a Wellness Unleashed: Empowering Women through Self-Care workshop I helped at:

1. I am worthy of taking time for myself and my well-being.
2. Nurturing my mind, body, and spirit is a priority, not a luxury.
3. I honor my journey and embrace my growth.
4. I am resilient, strong, and capable of overcoming challenges.
5. Every day, I choose to focus on the positive and let go of the negative.
6. I deserve love, compassion, and understanding, especially from myself.
7. I am in control of my happiness and create my own joy.
8. I listen to my body and give it the rest and care it needs.
9. I am grateful for my unique qualities and embrace my individuality.
10. I am empowered to make decisions that support my health and well-being.

Lastly, during the day, there are macro (for example, 10 minutes of intentional positive affirmations or meditation or prayer) and micro (for example, 1 minute or 1 second) moments. It will be important to stay positive during the many micro moments you have. That will be the real test and show your progress.

## Social Media

Self-awareness of your habits is important to implement change. What you consume daily is important to keep your mind positive. How can you start to change your mindset? By learning! Social media can be used for good if used for education. Curating your feed to show you positive and educational messages can help provide ideas and show you that you are not alone in your struggles.

## Past Trauma

Our mind cannot differentiate between the event and a memory of the event. Our body goes into a fight or flight state and it becomes a challenge to keep moving forward when we spend time looking into our past and having a victim mindset. However, when undergoing therapy that is a healthy way to process past trauma and figure out any triggers. With time, hopefully, we can start to heal and see that our past trauma was something that was done FOR us, not TO us. We will be able to heal and learn from it and grow. It is the difference between having a victim versus a growth mindset.

## Financial Independence

I believe that without a goal to become financially independent, it will be more challenging to embrace your female sensuality. When there is a lack of financial security, we lack the ability to nurture our mind, body, and soul easily and see it as a luxury instead of a priority. What does becoming financially independent mean? It is a work-optional lifestyle that still meets expenses and _____ (you fill in the blank/what is your ideal life?).

How are you going to gain financial independence? You will need a financial roadmap.

Check out: HowMoneyWorks - howmoneyworks.com/anam. In a nutshell, there are seven money milestones:

1. Financial Education
2. Proper Protection
3. Emergency Fund
4. Debt Management
5. Cash Flow
6. Build Wealth
7. Protect Wealth

## Imagination

Provide the universe with an order or demand about what we want by using your imagination. When we have a broad focus, we grow and find our solutions. When we have a narrow focus, we grow our problems because that is all we see. Take a bath, relax, and close your eyes, what do you see? What type of woman or life do you picture? Release that picture and start acting like you already have it. In a nutshell, you need to figure out what you want. If you don't know what you want, read *Rich As F*ck: More Money Than You Know What To Do With* by Amanda Frances. It is a life-changing book. My hope would be that you figure out what you want by opening your imagination without restraints.

## Maybe; This or Better Philosophy

Lastly, what is a maybe; this or better philosophy? It is a mindset where you are able to detach from outcomes by avoiding to label events as good or bad and instead labeling it "maybe" until more events unfold and believing that your life is great as is or it will be better. Think

Wednesday Addams, unfazed, confident, and clever. For example, if dating and the guy breaks up with you, avoid labeling said event as good or bad. Try labeling it as "maybe" instead and wait and see what happens as more events unfold. Next, believe that life is great as is and the next man you date will be better than the last. Either philosophy will help keep your mindset positive. Life is too short to feel miserable.

## Step 2: The Heart

When embracing our female sensuality and energy, we need to be able to feel our emotions, but not become them. It is okay to feel sad, but not okay to become sad and thus depressed. Life is too short to feel miserable. Tomorrow is not guaranteed. Our emotions are powerful and we need to be able to release them one way or another. So how do we process our emotions? You can practice the TDRRA system.

1. Trigger (what triggered my emotional outburst?)
2. Deep Breath (ground yourself; breathe in for two seconds and exhale for four or more seconds until you are calm)
3. Reflect with nonjudgment and self-compassion (analyze and take time to debrief the chain of events)
4. Release (let it go)
5. Action (example: tomorrow I will do better)

By taking the time to analyze your emotions, you can become soft and feminine on the outside and firm and secure on the inside. For example, when you wake up every morning, how do you feel? What is your baseline? Do you wake up happy, sad, grumpy, angry, or something else? If you wake up happy and there is a negative event, like getting cut off in traffic, how long does it take you to go back to baseline? 10 seconds, 10 minutes, or all day? If you wake up happy and have a 10-minute positive self-talk/affirmation or meditation, then look at yourself in the mirror, do you stay positive minute by minute, second by second during your day? These micro moments are important because that is a sign of your development and help you maintain composure when things do not go as planned. You will be able to embrace the positive concept/image of yourself and prioritize yourself without feeling guilty. Otherwise, we keep neglecting ourselves, being people pleasers, putting others first, and becoming resentful. After having a change in mindset, it will be easier to say "no" and set boundaries. The next step is to communicate what you want to yourself, your partner, your kids, and a higher power. Ask yourself, how can I love myself today or this week? Only you will know what you need. A daily practice I was recommended was journaling and answering two questions daily:

1. What was one thing I did for myself today?
2. What am I proud of today?

These two questions are short yet profound. They help you realize if you are putting yourself first or not. You cannot give from an empty cup. When I cannot answer the questions, I realize I did not do anything for myself. It does not have to be anything big like going to the gym. It can be small like doing your hair. Only you know what you need. Self-care is not selfish. It is self-love. Treat yourself, you deserve it.

## Step 3: The Soul

Whether you are religious or spiritual, whether you believe in God, another higher power, or the universe, we all look up to a power outside of us. Having a strong faith practice helps ground and center ourselves. It helps pay attention to your soul. Set an appointment with your higher power and pray or meditate for twenty or thirty minutes if you can. The amount of time does not matter as much as being disciplined to do it daily. Our soul wants and/or needs to express gratitude for the things we already have and learn to WANT the things we already have. For me, learning to want the things I already had was a game changer and helped me keep a positive mindset and perspective. Here are some affirmations that help with the soul. Fill in the underlined words with your own words:

1. I know it will all work out.
2. I trust in <u>the higher power</u>.
3. <u>The universe</u> always has my back.

## Step 4: The Body

## Environment

After all the inner work of the mind, heart, and spirit, comes the outer work of the body. Female sensuality like confidence or vulnerability needs an environment that helps foster it. Having the right people and physical environment matters because people can hold you back. You cannot change the personality of those people. Ask who you are with those people, friends, and family included. Ask if your location is conducive to your new juicy life. If needed, cut the toxic people from your life and move locations if you must. It is easier to find people in your same energy wavelength than trying to get people on the same energy wavelength as you.

## Health

You cannot do anything without health. If you do not feel good, you will not have the energy to do anything. If you are clinically depressed, it is a challenge to get out of bed. If you have a chronic medical diagnosis, you are limiting your quality of life. How you treat your body impacts how you treat your mind. Our body is a temple. It is the vehicle in which we explore and experience the world. Living a healthy lifestyle is key to having quality of life. For me, that means having the ability to be independent of my activities of daily living. It is something that we can control.

What does living a healthy lifestyle entail?

- Physical Relaxation - work with your body, not against it
  - o Tense/relax, progressive relaxation
  - o Massages
  - o Chiropractor
  - o Urinate often
  - o Freedom to move, drink, eat
- Physical activity (ex: walking, exercising, hiking, dancing, joining a gym)
- Nutrition (well-rounded diet, moderation, supplements, Herbally Grounded at herballygrounded.com)
- Hygiene (routines and natural products, for example, no aluminum deodorants)
  - o Natural products (for example, Doterra)

Additionally, if becoming financially independent is already a goal you are working on, it will make it easier to accomplish the activities recommended like having a gym membership, receiving massages, or going to the chiropractor regularly. Next, the more you prioritize your body, the better you feel in your own skin and have quality of life. In my personal experience, dancing was my life-saver. By dancing, I was having fun and working out, it was a two-for-one. The more types of dances I tried like salsa, bachata, pole dancing, or heels classes, the more comfortable I felt in my own skin. I was able to touch my body without shame, feel sensual, and feel confident doing so. I also started recording myself after every class. It was a way to monitor my progress and keep myself accountable to keep going to class. As a Certified Lactation Counselor, I have been surprised on more than one occasion how many women do not feel comfortable touching their breasts to monitor their breast tissue which is essential to avoid any breast clogs or worse, mastitis (an infection of the breast tissue).

## Routine

Creating a maintenance routine and signature look (think signature hairstyle and signature nails) for yourself is key to your female sensuality. For example, I need a pedicure every three weeks or at least once a month to avoid ingrown toenails. For my signature look, I curl my hair or in a time crunch, straighten my baby hairs alongside my forehead and put my hair in a ponytail. As a mom of three, doing my hair is my nonnegotiable to fill my cup, feel my best, and set a good example to my daughters of doing something for myself.

Moreover, we are not all born a natural beauty when we roll out of bed. We can all learn how to use our unique features and create our OWN standard of beauty and sexy uniqueness. We can create a maintenance calendar based on our self-attributes. It is smart to be able to roll out of bed a four or five out of ten and then put yourself together to look like a seven or eight out of ten. Ask yourself, what makes you look or feel hot? For example, I love eyelash extensions. One time the eyelash tech told me her job was to enhance women's beauty. I loved that! We are all doing our best to enhance ourselves and look our best. If you are having trouble, you can take make-up lessons (like I did) or find a modiste to help you figure out what type of clothes look best on your body. You can also create a daily routine and a quick routine for the days you do not have the energy to go all out.

## Dressing

What you wear is important. It is a nonverbal way to communicate to the world how you feel on the inside. There is a difference in wearing versus styling your clothes. There is an art in dressing. It is a way of self-love. Clothes are your friends and you learn to wear and style them for different occasions. For example, wearing baggy clothes versus wearing form-fitting clothes can make a difference in how you feel about yourself and your sensuality. Wearing sexy lingerie or pajamas at night for yourself even if you live alone is a wonderful way to express your confidence and feel good about yourself. The type of underwear you use although not seen can impact your daily life and bring sexiness. You wear clothes for yourself to impress yourself. There is a magnetic energy created when you dress to impress.

## Boudoir Photography

Taking boudoir photography is a great way to celebrate yourself and your body. I enjoy taking these types of photos because it is empowering to see myself as beautiful and sensual as any model, especially with a postpartum body of three. I highly encourage trying it out. It is fun and you will have tangible memories to see, especially on days when you have doubts.

## Conclusion

Understanding female sensuality is a journey. We are all at different times in our lives. These four steps can be done in the order described, in the order you find easiest to work on, or can be worked on simultaneously. There is no wrong or right way. What is important is your comfort level, investing in yourself, and developing your feminine sensuality, feminine energy, and becoming a high-value woman to live a life you are genuinely happy with. As a peer-to-peer mentor, I can help keep you accountable. Remember, you are worthy!

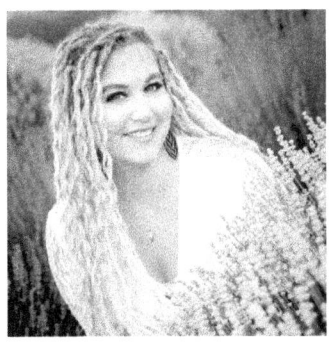

## Amber Lansdale

Amber Lansdale Coaching
Master Empowerment Coach

https://www.linkedin.com/in/amber-lansdale-89b2b2310/
https://www.facebook.com/profile.php?id=100065456141326
https://www.instagram.com/amberlansdale_coaching/
https://amberlansdale.com/

Amber has always felt destined to make a significant impact in this world.

Raised in Grand Rapids, MI, she constantly searched for her place, often feeling like the 'weird horse girl' who never quite fit in. Despite having many friends, she struggled to find where she belonged. Following the expected path, Amber spent years in college, ultimately earning a bachelor's degree specializing in Cardiovascular Sonography. As a Sonographer, she found satisfaction, but it was the deeper connections with patients that truly fulfilled her.

Amber's seemingly great life was fraught with challenges. She hit rock bottom in her late twenties, battling self-doubt, unhealthy relationships, and inner demons. During a low point, a coworker suggested coaching. Intrigued, Amber embarked on a journey of self-discovery, eventually becoming a certified master empowerment coach. Now, she empowers others to rewrite their stories, reclaim their power, and embrace lives filled with purpose, joy, and self-love.

# Breaking Free: Finding Authentic Sensuality

By Amber Lansdale

From a young age, we are taught by those around us how to act, what to wear, and who to be. Born pure and innocent, we initially have no knowledge of our true selves. As we grow older, we begin to develop our own personalities and start showing up in the world authentically. However, this process often gets disrupted by societal and familial expectations. We are told what is and isn't "appropriate."

As young girls especially, we receive constant directives on how to behave, what to wear, and how we should look and act. Phrases like "act like a lady," "big girls don't cry," and "you can't wear that, boys will get the wrong impression" are all too common. We are taught not to take up space and to keep our voices down because- "little girls are to be seen not heard."

Growing up, I heard all of these things. As I got older, my grandparents and other close family members were particularly hard on me. I would hear comments like "You're getting fat," "Are you pregnant?", "Boys don't like fat girls, you should watch your weight," and "You're too fat to do sports."

Hello, body-image issues and childhood trauma!

My body-image issues were often dealt with by emotional eating. I was extremely depressed on the inside. I always felt like the "fat" friend. Boys didn't like me, and I was never the first choice for a girlfriend. I frequently wore clothes that didn't flatter my body, just trying to fit in. I remember sneaking my hip-hugger jeans in my backpack to school because my mom would make me wear high-waisted pants that even my friends would make fun of me for.

As I got older, I became desperate for love and attention. My friends were all in relationships and I was not. I was willing to settle for anyone who would give me the time of day. My worth wasn't defined by my own perspective but by the perspectives of others. This led me to settle for relationships built on disrespect and manipulation. I remember losing my virginity to a boy who had dated all of my friends before he even considered dating me. He told me that if I didn't have sex with him, he would find someone who would. Desperate not to lose the only boyfriend I could get, I gave in. He later cheated on me multiple times, and I still stayed because I had zero respect for myself or my body.

As I reached my adult years, I carried all of my childhood traumas with me. I didn't love or respect myself and continued to choose relationships that mirrored this lack of respect. I clung to anyone and everyone who would give me attention. In my late twenties, I hit a breaking point. I was deeply depressed and weighed more than I ever had in my life. Despite multiple attempts to diet and workout, the weight wouldn't shed. I was completely disconnected from my body, and sex became a routine action to keep my partner happy; I didn't even enjoy it. I knew I had hit rock bottom when I found myself lying in the bathtub, crying uncontrollably, praying to cry myself to sleep and slip under the water to end all the pain.

Little did I know that breaking point would be my last. That same week, I was talking to a coworker about changing my career. She was transitioning into a career in life coaching and suggested I look into it as well. She said I had such a positive and inspiring personality and believed I would be great at it. This suggestion led me to start a women's empowerment certification course, which changed my entire life.

These courses led me through my own healing journey. I began doing the tough, deep work I needed to heal. I confronted and worked through all the shame and guilt I had been carrying and learned to love my body again. I realized I could demand respect, love my body just the way it is, and provide it with everything it needs and desires.

I discovered aerial fitness, which helped me find confidence and strength through a workout I genuinely loved and looked forward to. I started losing weight and feeling really good about myself. For once, I didn't feel like a prisoner in my own body. It truly is amazing, once we start loving ourselves from the inside our outside appearance also begins to change. We just naturally begin to carry ourselves differently.

I wanted to find a way to celebrate myself and my body. A good friend of mine introduced me to boudoir photography. After just one photo shoot, I was hooked. I saw myself in a whole new light. I wasn't a size two; in fact, I was a size 12 at best, but damn, I was hot. I began to love my curves, and seeing myself in boudoir photos made my self-confidence skyrocket. If you have never tried boudoir, I highly recommend it. Major confidence boost.

With this newfound confidence and love for my body, I learned that sex was enjoyable, whether it was by myself or with a partner. It became an act of pleasure that my body craved, no longer just something I did to keep a man around. In fact, I realized I didn't even need a man—sometimes it was even better without one! Unfortunately, I had to teach myself all of this, as sex wasn't really a topic I could discuss with my mom. Even in my twenties and thirties, she didn't want to know I was having sex. It's fascinating to me how sex remains a taboo subject for many. We're often sent out into the world to figure it out on our own. Sure, we have sex-ed to teach us about safe sex, but who is going to teach us about pleasure?

It was through my empowerment coaching that I learned about pleasure. I discovered that pleasure was a good thing and that I deserved it. My poor self-image had been holding me back. I had a bad relationship with myself, making it difficult to find pleasure. Before my newfound confidence, I thought pleasuring myself was gross. I couldn't enjoy sex because I was too worried about what I looked like. I didn't feel sexy, and that thought consumed my mind to the point where I couldn't even relax.

Through my experiences, I learned the importance of embracing sensuality as a natural and empowering part of being a woman. It was a journey of self-discovery and empowerment, where I had to confront societal norms and expectations and redefine my relationship with my body and desires.

Exploring sensuality became a catalyst for my personal growth and transformation. I discovered the interconnectedness of physical sensations and emotional experiences, learning to trust my intuition and honor my desires. Through practical exercises and guidance, I cultivated mindfulness and presence in my everyday life, allowing me to savor moments of pleasure and delight.

Overcoming shame and guilt was a significant hurdle on my journey, but I found strength in embracing sensuality as a source of empowerment and self-expression. I learned to prioritize pleasure as a fundamental aspect of self-care and well-being, indulging in sensual pleasures and rituals that nourished my body and soul.

Today, as a master empowerment coach, I specialize in guiding women through deep healing to cultivate self-love and rediscover their inner confidence. My mission is to inspire others to embrace their sensuality as a path to vibrant and fulfilling lives, celebrating the beauty and power of their feminine essence.

In my journey, I discovered that embracing sensuality isn't just about accepting and loving our bodies, but also about fostering curiosity, playfulness, and self-compassion. These elements are vital in creating a vibrant and fulfilling life.

# Curiosity

Curiosity is an invitation to explore our bodies and desires with an open mind. It's about being inquisitive and adventurous, allowing ourselves to experience new sensations and pleasures without judgment. When we approach our sensuality with curiosity, we break free from preconceived notions and societal limitations, opening ourselves to a world of possibilities.

Imagine a child discovering the world for the first time, with wide-eyed wonder and an eagerness to learn. This same sense of curiosity can be applied to our own bodies. We often overlook the incredible capacity for pleasure that our bodies possess, constrained by societal norms and personal insecurities. By fostering curiosity, we give ourselves permission to explore these capacities without fear or shame.

Curiosity in sensuality means taking the time to learn what feels good for you. It could be as simple as touching your skin with different textures—silk, fur, or even feathers—to see how each sensation feels. It might involve experimenting with different types of touch, pressure, and rhythms to discover what excites and soothes you. This exploration is not limited to physical touch but extends to all our senses. Try lighting scented candles to stimulate your sense of smell, or listening to music that moves you emotionally and physically. Every sense can be a pathway to deeper sensuality.

In relationships, curiosity can transform how we connect with our partners. Instead of assuming we know what our partner likes, we can ask questions, be observant, and try new things together. This not only keeps the relationship dynamic and exciting but also builds intimacy and trust. By being curious about our partner's desires and needs, we create a safe space for them to explore their own sensuality alongside us.

Curiosity also encourages us to explore our fantasies and desires without judgment. It's normal to have fantasies, and they can be a healthy part of our sensual lives. By allowing ourselves to explore these fantasies, either through imagination or discussion with a partner, we can understand more about what we desire and why. This self-awareness can lead to more fulfilling sexual experiences.

Moreover, curiosity helps us understand that sensuality is not confined to the bedroom. It can be integrated into our daily lives through mindfulness and presence. Simple acts like enjoying the taste of our food, feeling the warmth of the sun on our skin, or savoring the sensation of water running over our body in the shower can all be deeply sensual experiences. By being curious and present in these moments, we can enrich our daily lives with sensual pleasure.

Ultimately, cultivating curiosity in our sensual journey is about embracing an attitude of lifelong learning and exploration. It's about rejecting the notion that there is a "right" way to be sensual and instead discovering what is uniquely pleasurable and fulfilling for each of us. Through curiosity, we can unlock deeper levels of self-awareness, intimacy, and joy, transforming our understanding and experience of sensuality.

## Playfulness

Playfulness brings joy and lightness into our sensual experiences. It encourages us to engage with our bodies in a fun and carefree manner, transforming how we perceive and interact with our own sensuality. When we approach our sensual selves with a sense of play, we release the pressures of performance and perfection, allowing for a more authentic and enjoyable experience.

Consider the simple act of dancing. Imagine dancing in your living room, free from judgment and self-consciousness, feeling the rhythm of the music, the movement of your limbs, and the sheer joy of letting go. This liberating act connects us with our bodies in a joyful and primal way, heightening our physical and emotional pleasure.

Playful experimentation can also deepen our sensual experiences. Picture you and your partner blindfolding each other, taking turns to explore different sensations—feathers, ice cubes, massage oils, or even various fabrics. This playful exploration not only intensifies physical sensations but also builds trust and intimacy, turning sensual exploration into a shared adventure where both partners revel in each other's responses.

Laughter is another powerful element of playfulness that can transform our sensual experiences. Laughing reminds us not to take ourselves too seriously and to enjoy the present moment. Laughter releases endorphins, natural mood lifters that enhance the overall pleasure of our sensual encounters, creating a positive feedback loop where joy begets more joy.

Playfulness invites creativity into our sensual journey. It encourages us to explore new activities, positions, and fantasies without fear of judgment. Whether it's role-playing, trying out new lingerie, or setting up a romantic scavenger hunt, playfulness allows us to step outside our comfort zones and discover new facets of our sensuality. This creativity can reignite passion and bring fresh, exciting energy into our relationships.

Furthermore, playfulness helps us reconnect with our inner child—the part of us that is spontaneous, curious, and full of wonder. As children, we experienced the world with an open heart and an adventurous spirit. By tapping into this playful mindset, we can bring a similar sense of wonder and excitement into our adult lives. This not only enhances our personal pleasure but also enriches our connections with others.

Incorporating playfulness into our sensual journey also means giving ourselves permission to be imperfect. It's about embracing the awkward, the funny, and the unexpected moments that inevitably arise. Instead of feeling embarrassed or discouraged, we can choose to laugh and continue exploring. This acceptance of imperfection creates a more relaxed and enjoyable experience, where the focus is on connection and pleasure rather than performance.

Ultimately, playfulness in sensuality is about embracing joy and spontaneity. It's about creating a space where we can explore, experiment, and express ourselves freely. By infusing our sensual experiences with playfulness, we can rediscover the joy of physical pleasure, deepen our emotional connections, and enhance our overall well-being. It transforms sensuality from a routine act into a delightful adventure, filled with laughter, creativity, and profound joy.

## Self-Compassion

Self-compassion is the cornerstone of a healthy and positive relationship with ourselves. It means treating ourselves with the same kindness and understanding we would offer a close friend, especially during times of challenge or insecurity. By practicing self-compassion, we create a nurturing internal environment that allows us to embrace our sensuality without guilt or shame.

At its heart, self-compassion is about recognizing our inherent worthiness. It's about understanding that we deserve love, pleasure, and joy simply because we exist. This mindset shifts the way we view ourselves and our bodies, transforming our inner dialogue from one of criticism to one of acceptance and love.

When challenges or insecurities arise, it's easy to fall into patterns of negative self-talk. We might criticize our bodies, compare ourselves to others, or feel unworthy of pleasure. Self-compassion offers a powerful antidote to these destructive tendencies. It encourages us to acknowledge our imperfections and struggles without judgment and respond to ourselves with empathy and kindness.

Imagine a situation where you feel insecure about your body. Instead of berating yourself for not meeting societal standards of beauty, self-compassion invites you to acknowledge your feelings without harsh judgment. You might say to yourself, "It's okay to feel this way. My body is beautiful and worthy of love just as it is." This shift in perspective helps to break the cycle of negative self-talk and promotes a more positive and accepting view of yourself.

Embracing self-compassion in our sensual journey also means giving ourselves permission to experience pleasure. Many of us carry guilt or shame around our desires, often due to societal or cultural conditioning. Self-compassion helps us to recognize that our desires are natural and that seeking pleasure is a healthy part of being human. By treating ourselves with kindness, we can explore our sensuality without the burden of guilt or shame.

Incorporating self-compassion into our daily lives can profoundly impact our sensual experiences. When we treat ourselves with kindness and understanding, we create a safe space to explore our desires and pleasures. This compassionate approach helps us to feel more comfortable in our bodies and more open to intimate connections.

For instance, if we feel self-conscious about our appearance during intimacy, self-compassion allows us to acknowledge those feelings without letting them take over. We can remind ourselves that our partner is with us because they find us attractive and enjoy our company. This shift in focus from self-criticism to self-acceptance enhances our ability to be present and enjoy the moment fully.

Moreover, self-compassion helps us to set healthy boundaries and communicate our needs effectively. When we value ourselves and our well-being, we are more likely to advocate for our desires and ensure that our sensual experiences are mutually satisfying. This leads to more fulfilling and respectful relationships, where both partners feel valued and heard.

Ultimately, self-compassion is about embracing ourselves fully, with all our strengths and vulnerabilities. It allows us to approach our sensuality from a place of love and acceptance, rather than fear or judgment. By cultivating self-compassion, we create a foundation for a more joyful, authentic, and fulfilling sensual life.

As you embark on your own journey of self-discovery and empowerment, remember that sensuality is a multifaceted experience that encompasses physical, emotional, and spiritual aspects. By integrating curiosity, playfulness, and self-compassion into your life, you can cultivate a deeper connection with your body and desires, ultimately leading to a more vibrant and fulfilling life.

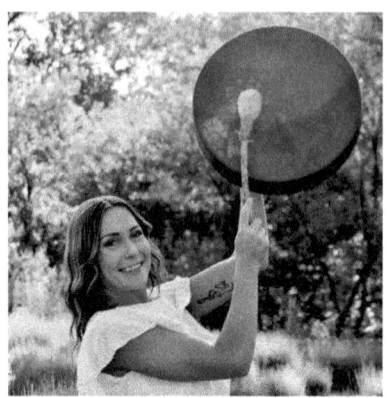

**Lindsey Pollock**

Transformational Advocate for Sound Design Healing

https://www.facebook.com/t.shorty08?mibextid=LQQJ4d
https://www.instagram.com/lindseypollock_/

An expert at helping connect with those who are ready to dive deep within being guided through to their authentic truth within knowing, feeling and embodying their innate sound of beat within a heart so Divine, pure for creating an environment where the empowering voice gives them the grounds to be rooted immensely in their purpose.

I am here to open the doors for the next chapter of my journey, becoming the best version of myself to share these beautiful moments with those seeking genuine self love through being aware, acknowledging and accepting parts that tend to veer a way forward - however truth will show up from the depths, and free on the surface.

I have the capacity to hold a safe, secure, stable and sane space for those ready to give + receive the same support.

# Golden Gate of Sacred Sensuality

By Lindsey Pollock

Heal thy mind.

Heal thy heart.

Heal thy body.

Heal with Spirit.

& FEEL your SELF!

What claiming my Sacred Sensuality, openly, within the bridge of awareness, acknowledging, and accepting has been wild.

Choosing me. Over and above all beliefs of my faith, being born into a community of believers, that covered a women's rite of passage of the essence every Goddess carries.

Seek. Ponder. Pray. Are the things I must do?

I did seek. The love for my body, in all waysides, as early as the age of 4. What I found was a deeper understanding that no one REALLY understands what their relationship with their body means, until they choose to explore the relationship within their own Divine Feminine and Divine Masculine connection.

That connection for me started in my own shadow, at the age of 29. The shadow of all the parts of me calling to be known, heard, seen, spoken, felt, creative, empowering, and supportive in the midst of the awakening of my inner self-conceptions of the female body, rejuvenating the feeling of physical, mental, emotional, spiritual, intellectual, and sensual energy craving for a warm, stimulating experience of pure cosmic bliss.

I began to invest in my body, seeking anything to activate those feelings welling up inside to be released in the pursuit of passion and the sweetness of love. I flew in so I could live in the moment, to be open for change, to pursue dreams with optimism, in all directions representing flexibility and freedom.

One thing I was grateful for was the opportunity I kept opening up by choosing me. However, this showed from the core perspective and rose to the level of sexual potency from a sensual relationship with self, energy, and combat excellence - that I once labeled as "hyper-sexual" only feeling well for healing my womb and that is immensely satisfying for the lack of activating ALL of the senses.

The hum for the sweet nectar was awakening and I felt that the hum of my voice would have made it more pleasant. Breathwork is a key factor when rising to levels of consciousness of being within your sensuality.

Oh, the hum that is oh so yum. When your body feels it and signals for the mind to connect and keep that breath centered deep and released. The flow of energy that emerges from the sacred canyons of euphoria tastes sweeter and grounding. Have you ever been shocked by an electric current that fills your body? The spark, the tingle, and the sensation. Mm.

In my upbringing, I heard the words, "Don't touch yourself, and don't touch others." Kissing and hugging even became nonexistent. I was meant for touch. I was meant to taste. Those were my senses when even shaking someone's hand, the brush of someone's shoulder, and it went deeper. The energy that carried me wanted to come alive, move, and dance to the rhythmic exhilarating sounds of a little voice screaming inside, "CONNECT WITH ME!"

The dance in sensuality has come in many forms for me through this awakening of my sensual nature. Music can shift me in more ways than

I can even express, but the codes of movement into my body are ever-changing in the way I hold my mind. Entering that divine trust of my inner sacred song with melodies and beats that touch my sensual being.

The question of whether or how I chose a direction also came into play when I was beginning to open myself up to the way I know, feel, and embody my inner voice.

I had to face honoring parts of myself and ones that were also present, but not seen, heard, or felt. I had to learn to give my body, mind, and spirit gratitude, and make offerings while cleansing the fruits of my flower, and the garden was filled, ready to be harvested.

Divine grace was showing up through this in my sacral healing through the cycles, balance, dreams, phases, goals, grounding, and my mind was also attempting to release the judgment within my physical wisdom and create stability.

That's when it shifted. I was guided to a place for harnessing my life force so intentionally through facing challenges with how others perceive me, navigating around the houses of myself, embracing the power that I had, taking a leap of faith, and prompting myself to have the courage for this sparking passion, really tapping into an element that burned through in all ways. Om. The red, emotional wisdom, regeneration, and trust I felt, filled with love, passion, and compassion. I was brought to life through voluptuousness in a sense I had yet to understand.

This is where I had to get more clear with this part, of course, because it was reflecting on the way I was thinking versus how I was feeling. Those two were meant to connect. Through seeking inspiration, finding ways to raise my energy to bring more awareness, and what my plan was for the goal, I had to find balance and be initiative to keep myself from learning and breathing. I felt like a little girl, which did exist within me, teaching myself new ways to open up what I was seeing and speaking up, and also on what was being created here for me. It was beautiful, yet, being an advocate for self is not one for the meek mind.

Parts were unraveling and I felt this impression come true for focusing inward. My body. My mind. Needed my spirit. Trauma was coming through, uprooting my ground. The locking of that cage made my body rest. For four months I lay in bed. Physical. Mental. Emotional. All opened up, connected, and guided me through a new phase of grounding. I was learning new health-related rituals. This one had me so deep. Being paralyzed by these things for so long had me crippled. Family. Friends. And close loved ones had to hear my voice in a new way. Many know, many had known. It was part of my childhood that brought me back to Mother Earth. The discovery I experienced, the logic within it all, and the mental wisdom I received created such a profound spiritual awakening and stability for me. Even through all the sorrow of real human truth.

Moments of connection through my sensuality, I had connections that shared deep, intimate encounters of their experiences that it was not quite an emotional response or attachment but more like a pay-the-fuck-attention message coming through. Expressions of, "It feels empowering, and regenerating a new and different space but not unfamiliar. It's like a reminder vibe. That is of the moon and all her cycles."

Which always led me to some natural realization of my deep roots. The ones that vessels kept having in comings and when those stroked those nerves. Oh, the flow of sensations. The merging of the body, mind, and spirit through these emotions felt at ease, once I learned to honor my womb in the woman I once was, the one I am currently, and the one I am becoming.

The rhythm of me is so eloquent, the way it flickers in every direction, simply drapes me in the reds, golds, and blacks of my eyes as if it were me in my body, mind, and spirit in such ways that sent glitter chills down one point, up another point in the sky of a world where there are so many stars, gleaming the spots that had been there all along, ready to be felt!

I learned at a later age the secret of my sensuality. The ways are infinitely there in the view, once you choose, it shows and the truth of your existence will always find its way. Where there is a level of endurance that you have to go through, really give in, and release your breath for the next stimulus cycle of sacred practice. I have so many beautiful modalities in these areas and there are little to none that I have chosen, given a whirl, and received healing.

Let's go with a version of me, where rhythm moves me, but add in lyrics, those become subliminal messages that I began to create with myself in dark ways and the harm I chose. With another energy reflecting harmful energy with themselves inside, then colliding with one another, exchanging all that dark energy, that's beaming with streams of consciousness placed in sacred sensuality is low. I have experienced and witnessed the knowing, feeling, and embodied that because I felt it was the only way. Self-affliction flew out, once I made a conscious effort to maintain peace with self-acceptance, that level of affection was infinitely better, for me. Because this is my story and my life. No energy can alter that, but me.

What gets the river flowing? How does this feel for you? I asked myself this in all ways. Cosmic? In what way? God-like? What is God? What piece can I use myself to get in touch with the source of my sovereignty as a human being? I've thought of it. I have done it. Yet, I have more questions asking myself to be even more honest and clear. Shivers, quivers, and tears have streamed through. From every angle. Tears from my physical body, from metaphysical tears, and the dance floor was filled with all eyes on me. Some juicy and some pure joy.

The body craves sex. The mind creates sensual awareness. The spirit holds sacred truths for this purpose of connection with one's self. Bridging all those gaps with sweet sounds is a taste, filled with a deep sense of belonging. Teaching these truths will help support the soul. Coming in with intentions of being able to express yourself in an essential way to opening up the heart. Letting go of shame, guilt, and fear within, shifts a feeling of security. My heart was destined to find love in me, lay those pieces all around me, as a lotus flower opens up and the rest is a new life spilling the seeds of my heart into the ground making those beautiful roots get deeper and give my dreams fruition from the darkness I use to dare to speak, at moments when I felt blocked in. Now I am free to voice all those chants, calling in what I have and being a voice by existing.

Have you ever felt robbed, until you found your way down a meadowland path that carried you to a pavement where you seamed the faults that were created deep beneath the earth and then lifted by a gust of air that whispered you into your breath that sent ashes wild, swirling and lifted a way deeper than you ever could know? Yum.

Sensuality sure changes as you choose more in. The incline of senses that once grounded you, to this nagging feeling that it is seeking a different form of attention and pleasure. How deep do I go with myself in this? It has gone, gone, gone and even beyond more than my body, mind, and spirit would ever know about if I had chosen to be scared of what is truly sacred. Om.G.

The feeling of swinging in with support, with the edges of my heart slowing down, as I exhale a breath, sinking into the sun-kissed embrace that makes my toes curl up and see the beauty all around me, flowing with the sounds of sweet dreams dripping from the sky. Those parts tickle my mind.

Static motion occurs when I breathe in a dream that I have been waiting to wake up in my mind and then realize that I have been resting in the cool dark place for a long period of my existence and the moment for almost a while now was transforming into the connection of my True Love.

There is one part of the mind that goes into several different motions for the pain relief that comes from what a body can experience. The more layers I begin to feel through, I know that I am creating this connection within to be a free spirit, as I am. It comes with asking myself, "Where is this coming from?" And at moments, I truly have to choose to release every breath that pauses, welling up tears in my eyes so that I can catch that sensation of well-being.

I will admit that I have been to the point where the low chords get hit with an overwhelming sense of how much more it can help me understand another piece in me that feels unknown, unheard of, and unfamiliar where I see myself as I am. I have to communicate with my dark shapes, which used to make me look like something I would rather find a better way to release. I did learn how to communicate with those shapes, but I also had to be comprehensively articulate in my own ways.

When I started this path of communication with the best parts of my sensual self, I had a new and unexpected understanding.

"What destructive patterns can I let go of?" and "What's my connection to the Divine, Source, Higher Consciousness; God?"

This was after a four-wall, body and mind had been built with stone, to withstand the fire that was always raging from the South and an air of North coming from above to clear the earth after the storm, a bright light ignited. It was magical.

I began to feel that I could not heal my relationship patterns by focusing entirely on other energies faulting and flowing over and over again. When I do align, while going inward, it means I take radical responsibility and am accountable for what actions I am willing to give, in order for change to occur.

Shadow work. Again. It isn't always pretty or easy. It requires that I do some deep inner exploration and take responsibility for how I show up in my relationships. The boundaries I set — route the ones I need more clarity on. The way I choose my behavior, expressing my emotions I have of myself, reflects in other parts of myself that I "punish" for past hurts. Ways I let my inner-child temper tantrum on the surface, when it needs nurturing from me and how I push buttons, testing moments and it can project itself into what's right in front of me. Those are heavy for me.

It's in my relationships with myself and bringing it home. Shadow work in relationships has an amount of courage and humility that is very much needed for opening.

Those versions do have these attributes that make you feel confident. Getting swept away in Universal Love can restore trust and harmony in relationships and it's encouraging when going through the process. Being so pure with one's heart can promote love, self-love, and compassion and create a deep inner healing and feeling of peace. It removes negative waves and streams in loving flows through your soul.

Healing is the union of opposing forces. There is no order for this. The integration of polarities and our understanding of creation in True unity, as oneness into wholeness that we are 🖤

Divine Love has conditions, but this can only mean in certain moments. The unconditioning where you meet your true love is in divine currency where you will know, feel and embody those conditions at the most conscious waking high. The inhale once taken of trauma, transmutes, and transcends, but only once the choice of truth exhales when you choose to be in complete authentic alignment with every piece of your experience is offered. It isn't a lifelong commitment. It has to show up and provide that love, to keep it, and it must be done with free will. Expecting nothing in return. This one can get tangled depending on where one's healing is happening, and how one is choosing to heal. When I love this way — I am offering my True Love — the vibe that allows all flow to be how they are for what they are. Continuously reassessing the relationship and deciding through the journey, if it is still aligning and it's given and receiving, freely.

Emit life in your mind.

Being sacred.

Being sensual.

Being sexual.

Those unions between your sacred, sensual and sexual points, have been in a constant state of constant confusion, conflict, and commitment for what I know of them, feel with them, and really encompass their relationship within me.

The moment I began living in my highest alignment was the moment the manifestation of those desires flowed in. Persist. Be disciplined, for yourself. Remain focused and watch how you quantum leap into your desired Divine Self of sacred knowledge that sensually allows you to become relaxed with your authentic sexuality.

Knowing thy Divine Nature has brought such profound changes in my existence. From being told it was, or had to be one way and knowing in my body, mind, and spirit that was far from my truth brought me through where I am now. I feel deeply inside the truth of my being as a human and as I move forward, it will only be a matter of awareness of my healing. I empathize with this feeling for myself and others who have shared their personal truths, and what we move through together, which reminds me how important it is to continue to align, share my own experiences, and help others through this process if they feel called to.

I am a believer in self-accountability and acceptance, those two, hand in hand have reigned supremely over my shift. In the shadows and in the light. I am enough, as I am.

You can say you know what something will be like until the experience comes and does its own correct course within you. For me, surrendering to those parts of my sacred soul, sexual desire, and sensuality will always remain in the heart of me. I will always have my kinks in my mind, but I have been given beautiful love to receive from the Golden Gate within to keep me guided from knowing what I was attached to, and releasing for the parts that I feel deeply rooted within to stay true.

That's how I found it. Letting go of the idea of something that I was attached to that was not mine to begin with and knowing, feeling, and embodying those parts of me that have always existed in Divine Love.

I will be creating a new course program through this and will be sharing. Grateful for my willingness to have faith in bringing myself home.

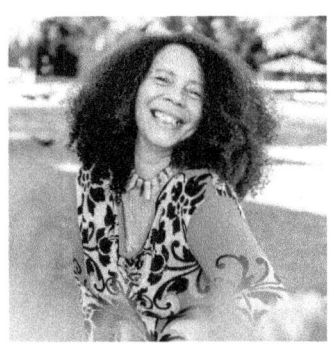

## Demetriah Annenayah

I AM POWERED BY LOVE
Sacred Feminine Coach

https://www.facebook.com/demetriahannenayah
https://www.instagram.com/iampoweredbylove
https://www.iampoweredbylove.live/
https://iampoweredbylove.com/

Demetriah Annenayah is a devoted advocate for the Sacred Feminine and a seasoned spiritual coach, empowering women to realize their true potential. With decades of experience in spiritual teaching, coaching, and energy healing, she has guided countless women on transformative journeys of self-discovery and manifestation. Her spiritual path began with surrendering to the Divine Creator, navigating personal trials, and gaining deep insights into spiritual growth. Drawing from the Source Creator and the Akashic Records, Demetriah integrates metaphysics, quantum physics, and soul technology in her unique guidance. Her vision is to awaken the Divine Feminine in every woman, fostering a world where women live authentically and powerfully. Her mission is to equip women with the tools and insights to overcome obstacles and manifest their dreams, leading lives of love, purpose, and fulfillment. Demetriah inspires women to embrace their spiritual power and create lasting change, becoming a beacon of empowerment and enlightenment in today's world.

# The Art of Sensual Healing and Pleasure of Sacred Union

By Demetriah Annenayah

Welcome, Sacred Sister! In this chapter, we'll explore the transformative power of sensuality, sexuality, and Samadhi by introducing you to the secret of Tantra, the gateway to love, intimacy, and money. Quick heads up: this chapter contains explicit language, sexual content, and a reference to an act of violence. Proceed with caution.

There are times when healing begins with the darkest moments. For me, that darkness started with a violent sexual trauma that shattered not only my body but also my spirit at the age of 12 years old. My scars and bruises were the curse and the blessing of my life. Those hidden wounds undermined my ability to harness love, sex, and money. By the age of 36 years old, I started to see what the damage was costing me: a non-reproductive womb, two marriages, and three failed businesses, plus the bonus of not being able to see people for who and what they were as bottom-feeding narcissists. My feelings of unworthiness and deeply ingrained beliefs kept me from achieving the success of my purpose, gifts, talents, skills, and abilities, as well as my dreams and desires. So, my life path turned into my Soul's purpose, fixing me. I just kept telling myself, "I am not broken."

My spiritual gifts and abilities were active at an early age—healing by touch, seeing visions, hearing messages, and sensing future outcomes. These gifts were my sacred connection to the Creator as if magically steering me toward a spiritual path. Yet, despite this connection, I remained isolated, lost, and disconnected from myself. God became my only refuge. My life, my Soul, and my sanity were quickly eroding through a plethora of addictions, bad decisions, and destructive friendships who enjoyed watching the shipwreck.

And, by the age of 37, I stood at a crossroads: Either I could let my trauma define me, or I could heal and reclaim myself. My warrior spirit would no longer allow me to live a broken, abandoned, and discarded life. I will make no illusions for you; I was at war. I wasn't sleeping with the enemy; I was the enemy. My life was a solitary confinement of pleasing everybody while never feeling safe in my body or at peace with my identity, constantly reflecting the expectations others had about my life, and worst of all, never being entirely able to engage in sensual and intimate experiences. Can you imagine?

So, for me, ambition was never about achieving external successes like wealth, love, or marriage. It was being genuinely self-made, not by the standards of other or societal beliefs or requirements, familial, cultural, or system structures. I was already my worst critic, so I needed to stand firmly on belief systems independently of anyone else's and dismantle all ideologies of who I once believed myself to be. Unknowingly, that drive and ambition allowed me to tear down ancestral and generational strongholds projected onto my life and the past life karma that had been imprinted on me. You may be ready to make these changes, too.

Shortly after my declaration from my divine intervention, I stumbled upon a Buddhist Temple offering an "Exploration of Tantra"; it was a two-year guided healing into self-discovery. A profound sense of peace enveloped me, so I signed up without hesitation. I discovered the connection between our bodies and the material world, and how our thoughts and feelings shape our reality. Each week, I focused on creating new mind-body connections, allowing me to align with my sacred feminine energy by utilizing my kundalini to balance abundance with my inner divine masculine energy.

# Understanding Sacred Feminine Energy in Kashmiri Tantra

In Kashmiri Shaivism, Sacred Feminine energy is revered as Shakti, the dynamic, creative force of the Universe. Kashmiri Tantra is a non-dualistic philosophy that sees the divine as a unified whole, where the masculine (Shiva) and feminine (Shakti) are inseparable and interdependent aspects of the same ultimate reality, Parama Shiva.

**The Sacred Feminine Aspects of Kashmiri Tantra:**

- **Shakti as the Dynamic Aspect of the Divine**: Shakti is the active, creative principle of life through divine expression, while Shiva represents pure consciousness of intelligence.
- **Union of Shiva and Shakti**: The ultimate goal in Kashmiri Tantra is to realize the union of Shiva and Shakti within oneself, which leads to spiritual awakening and liberation.
- **Embodiment and Empowerment**: The body is recognized as a sacred vessel, and practitioners explore the Divine within through embodied practices of sacred sexuality.

Over time, I was peeling back the layers of guilt, shame, and self-loathing, transforming my self-image and restoring my sense of worth. Each session required introspection, forgiveness, and a commitment to loving myself fully. It wasn't easy embracing sensuality and pleasure, shifting from self-sabotage to intentional living. Yoni Mapping was my lifeline to unlearning emotional states of being beyond self-sabotage, guilt, and shame. It helped to reimagine my body image, my physical appearance, and the lies I told myself about being ugly and unlovable. Yoni Mapping is a gentle yet powerful practice that allowed me to begin repairing my self-confidence through forgiveness and self-acceptance.

## Love Is a Consciousness and Not a Feeling

Yoni Mapping was vital in helping me restore my natural state of sensuality and passionate sexuality as a woman. In times past, I was struggling sexually and during moments of intimacy, battling with disassociation, detachment, lack of true pleasure, or sometimes numbness in my body during intercourse. It took me on a guided exploration of my Yoni, the 'sacred space' or 'source of all life.' I experienced a profound shift in consciousness as a woman connecting to her body for the first time.

So, when the thought occurred to me, "I no longer need to dishonor myself; I am the Sacred Feminine returning to its original sacred design."

I knew I was purging old wounds. You cannot put a price on internal peace and joy, and I can't tell you enough; it's fucking priceless.

It's not uncommon for women to struggle with the fear of vulnerability and intimacy, especially after enduring betrayals, heartbreaks, father wounds, and the imbalance of societal beliefs and the worldly limitations that many women face in trusting and being confident in their inner awareness, creative ability, and sovereignty. These traumas leave lasting emotional scars. The thought of opening up emotionally can feel terrifying, as it invites with it the risk of being hurt, rejected, or misunderstood. I, too, was once paralyzed by this fear; through the ancient wisdom of Tantra, I discovered that building walls around the heart, convincing myself it keeps others out, also keeps your love from pouring in.

These things invite low self-worth and negative self-beliefs through our internalized self-judgment, which can be crippling, blocking the flow of love and preventing women from creating the lives of love, intimacy, and money we desire. The repeated experience of rejection memorializes our sense of unworthiness, and these types of long-held convictions begin taking shape in our realities. It was my time to let go. Now, you can let go, too.

## Embracing Yoni

**Reconnect with Your Body:** Explore your body with mindfulness and compassion, developing a deeper connection and understanding of your unique anatomy.

**Release Emotional Blockages:** Gently touch and consciously explore your body to identify any blockages and work through them to release emotional pain and trauma.

**Cultivate Sensual Awareness and Pleasure:** Expand your capacity for pleasure by exploring what feels good, safe, and nurturing for your body.

**Empower and Reclaim Sovereignty:** Move away from external narratives of shame or control and toward self-empowerment, honoring their bodies as sacred.

Today, I utilize Yoni Mapping as a part of my Sacred Feminine Design to help women transform and release stored traumas, emotions, and blockages so they, too, can transform them. You see, through the Yoni Womb Healing I received, I gave birth miraculously at the age of 45 years old. Yoni Womb Healing restored my clinically diagnosed infertility; my withered ovaries and fallopian tubes back to life. So, I know all too well that stored emotions can create energetic blockages in the body and affect your ability to manifest love, sex, and money. Is it time for you to embrace what's yours?

## Practice Makes Perfect Tantric Samadhi Embodiment

I'd added another year to my Tantric Journey to engage at the practitioner level so that I could become an instructor of Kashmiri

Tantra. I wanted to give the gift of sacred feminine energy, Shakti, to other women to assist them in awakening their inner divinity. The past year of healing allowed me to walk away from a toxic relationship and recommit my vows to God. Plus, I noticed that my spiritual gifts and abilities had heightened and expanded, and my Soul's Purpose was becoming more soul-aligned with my purpose of helping other women align more fully with their own Soul's contract and lead them to their own Samadhi fulfillment with Source Creator.

Each teaching and healing invited me to question everything I believed or once thought true about myself and how I interacted with the world I was co-creating. The invitation was clear in my heart: Tantra was the portal to true intimacy with God. Submission and surrender are the access points of the Sacred Feminine Design because these dispositions provide us the portal to vulnerability, trust, and authenticity, pathways to true emotional intimacy so that we can create a Samadhi Sacred Union, which is something one could never treat as a transaction.

1. **The Sensual Supreme Consciousness of Samadhi:**
   - **Attainment:** In Kashmiri Shaivism, Samadhi is the state of being fully merged in divine consciousness and experiencing infinite bliss.
   - **Living:** Natural enlightenment is achieved when this realization is integrated into daily life through continued discipline and awareness of this divine unity.
2. **Embodiment of Sacred Feminine Consciousness:**
   - **Integration of Spiritual Realization:** After achieving Samadhi, the practitioner embodies the qualities of the divine consciousness of both masculine and feminine into their everyday lives by living in harmony with the Universe, radiating compassion, wisdom, and love, and positively contributing to the world around them.
   - **Continual Practice and Deepening:** Even after achieving Samadhi, practitioners continue their spiritual path and

practices to deepen their understanding and experience of divine unity, continuously aligning with the sacred feminine energy (Shakti) as the dynamic expression of the divine.

## Sex Is Not a Weapon

As I continued to grow in my Tantric practices, I learned of its ancient wisdom beyond the oneness with self but the dynamic intentions of conscious-based relationships with others. I often recalled that I traded myself to please others within my relationships because I didn't know who I was; I tried to be what I thought would make them love me. This type of dynamic makes the partner feel like they aren't being seen or appreciated, and, in turn, they might withhold that part of themselves from the other partner to receive the acknowledgment of their giving.

At this stage, partners intentionally engage in sensual intimacy rituals to align their energies. By using tantric techniques to optimize their frequency and exchange energy, they can experience a deep sense of unity and connection. This allows them to synchronize and move together as one, anchoring each other on a soul level and in physical reality and leading to greater prosperity through their shared purpose.

Synchronicity and harmony (The Samadhi Effect) can only occur through Kundalini activation in both partners during sexual intercourse. It only takes one partner to awaken and shift the other to an awakened state. In this sacred space, partners experience a merging of energies, where boundaries between 'self' and 'other' blur as they melt into desirous passion together beyond the realm of beds, rooms, bodies, and pleasure to experience the expansion and connection with Source Creator and the accessing of their joint soul purpose and union between the two individuals.

The essence of Samadhi within a relationship is a state of oneness in which both partners transcend their individuality and experience themselves as one unified being with two individual forms of self-mastery to embody and manifest their joint mission. This elevated state of bliss begins to flow in every avenue of their lives more and more effortlessly creating the ecstasy of their lives together.

## The Secret to a Sensual Samadhi Sacred Union

Sensual pleasure will provide the partnership more stimulation because of the energies weaving between the two. Not to mention, the sensual pleasure is out of this world. The more they surrender themselves to the freedom to experience nirvana through one another, the more Samadhi becomes a seamless exchange between each partner's strengths, wisdom, and unique gifts that are magnified by each other. Here, the union becomes a sacred force by transcending old roles, relationship rules, societal norms, and previously held expectations through Samsara. The sensual pleasure intensifies the purification of Samsara, and naturally occurs during their physical engagement which allows them to amplify their manifesting potential, individually and together, so they may be more fully soul-aligned with their divinely ordained mission with a bankroll to boot.

## The Role of Tantric Samadhi in Joint Soul Purpose

You can achieve a sacred union of oneness with your partner and approach your relationship with intention, openness, and a commitment to spiritual growth and healing as the reason for your relationship; no hidden agendas or motivation can be present in the purity of the light. Here are a few basic steps:

1. **Create a Sacred Space**: Set aside dedicated time and space, ensuring your space is free of distractions so you can concentrate on one another and the spiritual work.

2. **Engage in Regular Tantric Practices**: Incorporate sacred tantric touch with the suggested hand placements to honor Lingam and Yoni. These practices help align your energies and deepen your connection.

3. **Communicate Openly and Authentically**: Honest, open vulnerability is the only foreplay that will stir it up! Creating a sacred container of non-judgment deepens trust and emotional intimacy.

4. **Embrace Vulnerability**: Allow yourself to be vulnerable with your partner, sharing your innermost thoughts and emotions. This openness creates a powerful bond and facilitates a more intense healing and connection.

With the guidance of an expert, you can give your relationship more direct access to divine alignments and assignments so that you both can begin manifesting your sacred soul mission. This is how matches are made in heaven. You don't have to wait for your Twin Flame to show up in your life to evolve your relationship. Who wants the headache of a Twin Flame Union when you can heal your relationship and surpass the Twin Flame experience of being one soul instead of being two individuals with one mission?

## The Reverence and Arousal of Yoni Puja

After two years of embodiment and another year of instructor training, I became a Sacred Feminine Tantric Teacher, Guide, and Instructor. I was honored with a Yoni Puja Ritual and Ceremony, marking a new beginning for me. In Kashmiri Tantra, the Yoni is revered as a symbol of sacred feminine energy and the source of all life, and the Yoni Puja is a deeply personal and liberating ritual celebrating the sacred feminine within oneself or one's partner.

1. **Preparation and Setting Intentions**: Create a sacred container for your ritual and ceremony. Set a clear intention for awakening or activating your sacred feminine connection to embody.

2. **Grounding and Centering**: Begin with breathwork and meditation to ground yourself and connect with your body, focusing on deep, mindful breathing.
3. **Physical Cleansing and Anointing**: Gently cleanse the yoni area and anoint yourself. I developed a Sacred Ceremonial Blend called Sacred She.
4. **Offering Devotional Items**: Place offerings around the sacred space and recite affirmations or chants that honor the divine feminine and the Yoni.
5. **Yoni Worship**: Explore your Yoni with a gentle, loving touch, focusing on its beauty, power, and sacredness.
6. **Invocation of Divine Feminine Energy**: Invoke the presence of the divine feminine through invocation and prayer, asking for guidance, healing, and awareness.
7. **Closing the Ritual**: Conclude with gratitude, grounding, and a final blessing prayer, reflecting on the experience and integrating the energy shifts into your daily life.

## Sensual Samadhi: A Real-time Manifestation—My Tantric Testimony

It was a year after I completed my Tantric Certification when something miraculous happened: I met someone, or he landed on my life path. Kismet, Serendipity, Destiny, or Vertex—whatever you want to call it, I knew I was having a significant life path shift. I met this gorgeous man, and from across the aisle, he spoke to my body, although he hadn't even noticed me.

I responded on reflex, seizing the opportunity to get closer to him. The surge of sexual tension was unlike anything I'd ever experienced before. Although we hadn't consummated it, I knew it was a Samadhi experience. So, I graciously invited him to take the empty seat next to me. My newly found confidence became raging hormones overtaking my body. I'd never felt so enlivened; it was intoxicating.

My kundalini was rising, thrashing inside me; instinctively, I placed my rested hand on his upper thigh to complete the connection from his energy. The vortex of him sent me immediately into an astral projection into Samadhi. I was enraptured and no longer present in the material world; it was everything they described; it was happening! Yet, without the sexual penetration. They never mentioned anything about this. But I surrendered to every sensation because all I knew was I had to have him sexually to complete the process. After all, I was about to implode.

Yes, initially, I was selfishly consumed by him with my sexual agenda to prove that healing had occurred. My Tantric training gave me a different path—a safe container to trust myself and confront the fears racing through my head. I had to know, "Could I have sex with a complete stranger and connect with myself without shame, fear, and over-analyzing?" Was my curse broken? Could I find happiness? Was love a possibility? Could I be successful at God's calling for my life's purpose? Could I be in the moment and surrender myself to pleasure? So, before he could exit to leave, I made a bold and brazen blurring out to him, "I want to fuck your brains out."

I was astonished at the words falling from my mouth. It was so overt of me. Mind you, we'd just met, and of all places, a bar. Although the pick-up line was customary for bar activity, it was way out of my character. So much so that my friends jumped to my rescue, or it could have been jealousy. Unaware of what was happening, I knew they needn't worry. He had activated me, and I was in the throws of a Samadhi experience with him in the crowded bar while my friends watched the Super Bowl.

Yes, healing transformed many things about me, including the sexual trauma part. I knew the Samadhi was unfolding in real-time, so I could witness myself unfolding; the man was what you might call a manifestation. The real teaching of manifesting is this: to become, you must do, act, and experience your transformation by embodying the new energy of your manifestation process. Otherwise, how will you know you have succeeded? My life path was shifting on tectonic plates, and my entire body trembled with the adrenaline rush. That's when I heard, "Surrender to him."

Later that evening, I found myself at his house; I heard the channeled message repeated, "Surrender to him." So, I relented from my quest of self-satisfaction for obedience and complied with a Source Creator directive. So, instead of an ego-based mission, I understood the assignment was to recapture the Samadhi for us both. Although I wasn't the woman I am today, I submitted myself to him entirely. The knowledge I went there seeking to verify my self-confidence and fear of intimacy had been granted most beautifully. I felt no shame or fear in so doing.

Sitting in the dark, I was turned on by my confidence. I was looking for something other than the exit or an escape route. I wasn't anxious or paranoid. Then I heard, "He needed to be made whole and reclaim his sovereignty."

Again, Samadhi is about the soul contract between two people and their individual highest purpose. Only then can those two people provide a safe container for their continued personal growth and advance their purpose without the clingy need for a relationship. They will establish a holy, purified relationship called Sacred Union. It is the cocoon of light where the Creator nourishes each counterpart to prepare them for the future mission. It is here, beyond words, that the people's bodies anoint one another with consent to create a sensual seduction to eradicate their fears, embrace vulnerability, and step into a new reality of love and healing.

Although I didn't know the man, I had already fallen in love with his soul.

That night, as our bodies enmeshed into oneness, I felt safer than I had my entire life. It was the relief I needed. Every cell in my body quickening and tingling with exhilaration. It wasn't he who freed me; I freed myself, but he allowed me to experience loving the being inside of my skin. Together, we Samadhi'd, and I never wanted it to stop. I could feel him like I'd never felt with a man before.

The next day, I experienced no guilt or shame. This was uncommon. I also didn't have the usual codependent thoughts about what happens next or whether he likes me. I felt like a new person who no longer cared about these things and didn't dwell on them like I used to. I wasn't imagining a relationship with him or wishing he knew more about me. I didn't have any of the typical desires for attachments or codependent responses or possess any of my old behaviors. However, I did crave the connection, so I always wanted to be with him—it was from an empty place of neediness but of the liberty I had in enjoying my spiritual experience, even though he never knew.

As I honored and treasured him over the next four years, each time our souls intertwined sensually, I would receive specific messages about my lover regarding the man he was destined to become. I sat in quiet observance, watching him imbue his gifts, skills, talents, abilities, and education to create a new vision for his life. Serving him like I was taught was my sacred service. He poured into me in ways I could never explain to him; remember, spirituality wasn't a marketable commodity in 2009. So, discussing openly or assuming others would comprehend didn't feel appropriate. I remained quiet, fearing he would think it was some "voodoo, magic spell." None of which I would ever partake in. Although I poured into him, giving him what he deserved as a sacred masculine, my adoration, attention, and affection for my gratitude and appreciation for the gifts he bestowed upon me and the talents, skills, and abilities his soul guided me to embrace. So, there was a Samadhi exchange. Even though I still struggled to embody my Soul's purpose back then and how it enmeshed with me, he was the fire that ignited me to lean into it with full vigor.

The Samadhi was getting stronger between us as our gifts, skills, talents, and abilities began to increase synchronically. I started receiving telepathic thoughts and messages, and he began entering my dreams with private messages. For example, once, I misplaced my phone and was without it for ten days. He appeared in my dream shouting, "Where are you!" But, when his business took flight, landing a one million deal out the gate, I knew he was benefiting from the Samadhi too. I watched him intensely over the next four years as we continued our sensual Samadhi dance. He taught me things he was unaware I was learning; this is Samadhi. My business ventures increased in revenue and opportunities just by taking ownership of the Samadhi experience, fulfilling the joy and pleasure of our path wholeheartedly. It was weaving a rapturous thread of soul-activating growth into our lives. To this day, I remain in consecration to him. There can never be a second, third, or fourth Samadhi Union. It isn't designed for mass consumption or partner hopping. It is holy and sacred. And, yes, we're still together, having crazy insane intimacy and ramping up the next version of our co-purpose.

## Your Sacred Feminine Evolution Awaits

As you journeyed with me through my story, what areas of your life call for renewal? Is it expansive, soulful love? The desire to experience true intimacy and fulfillment? Perhaps it's sensual money and financial seduction you seek to embody? Or a soul-aligned business you are being called to create?

Through the ancient wisdom of Kashmiri Tantric secrets shared in this chapter, you have the tools to clear away the blockages that have held you back and to step boldly into a life filled with passion, purpose, and prosperity. Let me be your guide to help you apply these teachings to your daily life. Allow them to guide you in creating new, healthier experiences that resonate with your true self so that you can experience your own Samadhi.

To begin opening your internal sensual inferno as the Sacred Feminine, below are three powerful mantras dedicated to the goddesses of Kashmiri Tantra. These mantras are spiritual tools that align you with sacred feminine energies, helping you invoke their blessings and manifest their qualities in your life.

**Take a moment to breathe deeply and center yourself. Reflect on these questions:**

- What would it look like to truly embrace my Sacred Feminine energy?
- How can I cultivate a deeper connection with myself and my partner?
- What practices can I begin today to clear blockages and invite more love, joy, and abundance into my life?

As you ponder these questions, know that the path of Tantra is not just a journey—it's an invitation to weave the power of manifestation through truth on every level of your being, that 'something' you always thought was missing. Allow each question to stir your senses, activate your imagination, and entice you. Take a deep breath, center yourself, and open your womb. These Goddess Mantras are from the secret vault of my Sacred Feminine Design. Each mantra invokes the divine qualities of a different goddess by infusing her sovereignty with your energy to uplift, support, and assist you in beginning this journey with me.

## Parvati Mantra for Love and Devotion – Love

- *Mantra:* "Om Parvatyai Namaha"
- *Meaning:* This mantra is dedicated to Goddess Parvati, the goddess of love, devotion, fertility, and strength. Parvati embodies the energy of unconditional love and the nurturing aspect of the divine feminine.
- *How to Use:* Chant this mantra to strengthen your relationships, deepen your devotion, and cultivate qualities of compassion and love. It is particularly effective for fostering harmony in marital relationships and for personal growth in devotion. While chanting, imagine a soft pink light flowing from your heart, representing Parvati's unconditional love, spreading throughout your body and radiating outward, enhancing your capacity to love and nurture.

## Saraswati Mantra for Wisdom and Knowledge – Sex

- *Mantra:* "Om Aim Saraswati Namaha"
- *Meaning:* This mantra is a salutation to Goddess Saraswati, the goddess of wisdom, knowledge, music, and the arts. Invoke her blessings for wisdom, intellectual strength, and creative abilities.
- *How to Use:* Chant this mantra during meditation or study sessions to seek Saraswati's guidance for clarity of thought, wisdom, and knowledge. Visualize a white light emanating from the center of your being, representing the purity and clarity of Saraswati's wisdom, filling your mind and heart with knowledge and insight.

### Lakshmi Mantra for Abundance and Prosperity – Money

- *Mantra:* "Om Shreem Mahalakshmiyei Namaha"
- *Meaning:* This mantra is a prayer to Goddess Lakshmi, the goddess of wealth, fortune, and prosperity. "Shreem" is

considered a powerful seed sound (bija mantra) that attracts abundance and blessings.

- *How to Use:* Recite this mantra to invoke Goddess Lakshmi's blessings for financial prosperity, material wealth, and overall well-being. It is often chanted during rituals, before starting new ventures, or when seeking financial stability. As you chant, visualize golden light radiating from your heart, filling your surroundings with abundance and prosperity, inviting wealth in all its forms into your life.

Incorporating these mantras into your meditation and daily practices will invoke the divine blessings and energies of each Goddess—Saraswati, Lakshmi, and Parvati—into your life. Whether you desire love, sex or emotional intimacy, or money, these mantras serve to set the beginning stages of your sacred feminine evolution into your original design.

## Your Sacred Feminine Journey Awaits

You've been waiting for this moment, searching for answers, hoping for change, and feeling stuck in a cycle of unfulfilled relationships and missed opportunities. Here's your crossroad. Don't wait for change to happen—succumb to it. Imagine a life where you feel deeply connected to yourself, confident in your worth, and capable of attracting the love, intimacy, and financial freedom you deserve. Allow the forbidden and the hidden parts of you to be unearthed.

With over two decades of experience, I know firsthand how to guide others into creating the most pleasurable new life experiences and ecstasy because we all want a manifestation of something greater each time we do it. As a devoted advocate of sacred feminine rising, I will lead you to yours. With my experience as a Sacred Feminine Tantric Instructor, Guide, and Teacher, I have helped countless women activate a soul-aligned life with love, sex, and money.

This isn't just another program—it's your pathway to living a passionate life, where you know exactly who you know you are, and you're not afraid of creating it on your terms because there's nothing sexier than owning your power.

You're at the intercession—no more waiting for a miracle. This is your invitation to step into a new reality. Enrollment for the next season has already begun. Discover your true Sacred Feminine Design and achieve the soul-aligned Samadhi with your love, intimacy, and financial security. The enrollment window is closing soon. Visit the website for details.

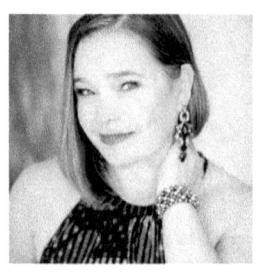

## Sylvia Becker-Hill

Founder of Becker-Hill Inc.

https://www.linkedin.com/in/sylviabeckerhill/
https://www.facebook.com/sylvia.beckerhill/
https://www.instagram.com/sylviabeckerhill/
https://becker-hill.com/
https://fenixtv.ap

Sylvia Becker-Hill is a true Renaissance woman, a 13-times published bestselling author, and a seasoned edutainer who has empowered thousands of corporate executives, women leaders, and entrepreneurs around the world since 1997.

In 2002, she became the first German coach to earn the coveted title of Professional Certified Coach from the International Coach Federation, establishing herself as an industry-shaping pioneer in the coaching world.

Her impressive educational background boasts two university degrees, while her portfolio showcases over 30 certifications in various change modalities, including her accreditation as one of the world's first 10 Certified Master Neuroplasticians in 2023.

Through her online TV show FLIP it! Sylvia is on the mission to empower you with all the knowledge, tools, and lasting transformation you need to "FLIP" everything that bothers, hurts, or blocks you from living your dream life into unquestionable Freedom, unconditional Love, envisioned Identity, and impactful Power.

Are you ready to feel unabashedly alive and powerful?

# FLIP Societal Shoulds Into Sensual Pleasure

By Sylvia Becker-Hill

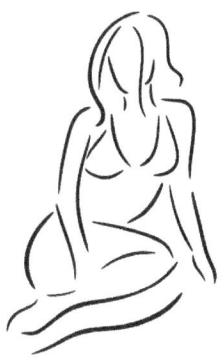

*"A woman who knows how to use her sensuality intentionally can't be fooled. She is the sovereign of her life."*
—*Sylvia Becker-Hill*

Most people, when hearing the word "sensuality," quickly jump to "sexuality." Though both are intimately connected, they are not the same. To liberate the latter, one must first understand the former.

To grasp words fully, we need to explore their historical usage and the meanings societies attributed to them. The word "sensual" in the title "Sensual Symphony" originally had a **negative tone** in the 15th century, being synonymous with "carnal," "relating to the flesh," "libidinous," "lascivious," "lecherous," "lustful," and "bodily." It contrasted sharply with "spiritual," which had positive connotations.

From this historical tidbit, one can sense how the word "sensual" evolved into society's efforts to suppress women's sensuality as sinful, viewing it as a **dangerous gateway to sexuality**.

Please stay with me on this path, even if it feels "too linguistic" (I studied linguistics for four years in Germany and can geek out on it).

You may not yet see how this will help liberate your sensuality from society's "shoulds," but we need to establish a shared understanding first. You might be amazed at what you'll discover through linguistics!

The root syllable "sens" in sensual and sensuality comes from the Latin word "sentire," meaning "to feel." "Sensus" encompassed feeling, thinking, and meaning! **The word "sense" originally meant "meaning."**

Feel into these definitions! Can you sense—pun intended—how important these distinctions are?

In modern times, we use "senses" to summarize all organs and capabilities that provide **information from our perception**:

1. of the external world (the classic 5 senses: seeing, hearing, tasting, smelling, touching)
2. from our body in relation to the external world (sensing movement and balance)
3. from within our body, known as "interoception."

Different cultures recognize different senses. In the English-speaking world, the 6th sense refers to "nonphysical perception skills" like intuition, anticipating the future, or remote viewing. The key points for this chapter are:

A. **Sensuality pertains to our bodies and their senses, allowing us to perceive important information.**
B. **Our senses empower us to make sense of and give meaning to our experiences.**
C. **Although the modern usage of "senses" is neutral, the old negative connotations persist subconsciously and somatically.**

In this chapter, we will explore:

1. Why knowing and using your senses intentionally is empowering and liberating.
2. How our senses and sexuality are connected.

3. Why society fears feminine sensuality and tries to contain, oppress, or suppress it.

4. How you can FLIP "Societal Shoulds" into "Sensual Pleasures."

## From Hermione to Aphrodite
## Why Knowing and Using Your Senses Intentionally
## Is Empowering and Liberating

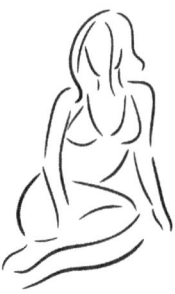

*"I was born into an ocean of pain and fears.*
*It was too overwhelming and scary, so I disconnected from my*
*body and its senses.*
*Like the fish that doesn't see the water it swims in, I thought*
*how I lived was normal.*
*I didn't know something was 'off' until it nearly killed me."*
*—Sylvia Becker-Hill*

I grew up in Germany in the late 60s and 70s with my mom, dad, and my maternal grandparents. All four struggled with undiagnosed, untreated trauma and PTSD from World War II, during which they were refugees, experienced starvation, faced life-threatening dangers, and witnessed horrors.

I was born into this family as the only child and became their "sunshine," their light. My young brain didn't understand what was going on, nor did I know until recently the full impact of intuitively caring for four struggling adults when I needed nurturing myself.

The mood of doom in our dark house, combined with the vow of silence over the painful past and the uptight conservatism of my Roman Catholic grandmother—who never dried her underwear in the garden because it was "not decent"—suffocated me. I was painfully lonely, learned to read by age four, declared books my best friends, and retreated from my body and the onslaught of painful emotions into my mind and intellect.

For most of my life, I lived like Hermione—Harry Potter's brilliant friend—feeding my head with books, taking my body for granted, and not using my senses consciously.

My passion for visual art and enjoyment of sexual exploration in my twenties opened the door to rediscovering my body. Yet, it took nearly thirty years of working as an executive coach and searching for powerful methods to help people change, combined with my body nearly killing me and a sabbatical from burnout, to truly discover the beauty, magic, and power of our senses.

We live in a time of high stress, while anxiety spreads like a virus, and societally conditioned busyness and dopamine addiction from social media are soaring. Many people—especially the newest generation, who grew up playing with screens instead of outdoors—live disassociated from their bodies. This leads most to **try to think themselves into a better mood** through "positive thinking," "repeating affirmations," or "silent meditating." Though beneficial, these methods are not as quick or powerful in calming your nervous system as using your own sensuality to lower cortisol and blood pressure, slow your heartbeat, and find calm in the midst of constant disaster news! Plus, you could—like I did for years!—think positive, meditate, and use powerful affirmations and still get killed by the impact of stress you don't know about—like it nearly happened to me!

# Finding Calmness in the Eye of the Storm
## - A Sense of Touch Exercise –

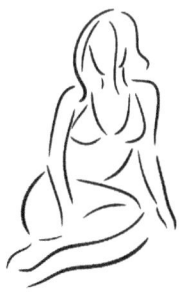

*"We curate ourselves unconsciously or intentionally
by what we repeatedly do. It is our daily habits that form us."*
—Sylvia Becker-Hill

Think of something bothering you right now, something that stresses or makes you anxious. Use your attention to go inward and scan your body. Where do you sense the stress or anxiety? How does it manifest? Tightness? Vibrating? A hole in your solar plexus? Dry mouth? Sense it! This is **interoception**: gathering information from inside your body.

Now, let's use your **sense of touch** to change your state. Roll up your sleeves to expose your lower arms, or if that's not possible, use your cheeks. Gently touch the inside of your left lower arm (or your left cheek) with the fingertips of your right hand. Do it slowly and lightly, like a feather. Breathe gently and slowly, then switch hands. Now, use the fingertips of your left hand to touch the inside of your right lower arm (or right cheek). Slow down and fully sense the sensations where you touch your skin. Notice what else this "heavening" exercise impacts.

**Simple touch exercises** activate the calming power of your "touch sense." Yet, you can use all your senses with full attention to become present and calm. For example, **listen** to quiet, meditative music, birdsong, ocean waves, or the wind. **Taste** a fresh fruit or a piece of chocolate, chewing slowly. **Smell** roses, freshly cut grass, hot herbal tea, or freshly baked bread. **See** a colorful painting, a dramatic sunset, or a wide-open landscape.

**The key to "sensual calming" is to do it slowly, without distractions, and with full focus on interoception—using felt sensations from the body's senses rather than projecting thoughts from your mind.** Remembering how a rose smelled is not the same as actually smelling it in the moment.

Here's an example of how I use my senses to shift myself and curate who I am: Yesterday, I felt restless in my office. I couldn't focus and didn't know what to tackle first from my long to-do list. I went into my art studio. I looked at my current painting and used the "sense of seeing" to switch my mood. Strong colors always uplift me. Then I sat down in the open door, closed my eyes, and used my "sense of hearing" to connect with my environment and the present moment. I heard birds in the pepper tree, children's laughter, and a motorbike passing by. I became so focused that all the sounds felt as if they were happening inside me. I felt ONE with my environment. **Those "sensual moments" not only calm my nervous system but also give meaning to my life.** I opened my eyes, stretched, and returned to my office, clear about what to tackle next.

This is what it can look like to use your sensuality intentionally to empower yourself!

## All Senses Are a Door to Arousal and Pleasure

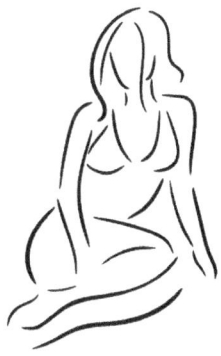

*"We are not human beings seeking spiritual experiences.*
*We are spiritual beings seeking human experiences."*
*—Teilhard de Chardin*
*(French Catholic priest, philosopher, and scientist)*

Metaphorically speaking, I believe all Gods envy us humans our bodies because of our senses. Only because of our body and senses can we smell the pheromones of a suitable partner and become aroused. Only because of our senses can we enjoy touching our beloved's body, our own skin, or that of our child. Only because of our eyes can we feel our heart beating faster when we see the person of our desire, admire our beautiful breasts, or see our reflection in the mirror wearing a gorgeous dress we just gifted ourselves. Only because of our clitoris, with over 10,000 nerve endings, can we fall into orgasmic, cosmic, ego-dissolving unity and wordless pleasure. Without our senses, humans wouldn't have discovered procreation through sexual intercourse, and the species would have died out. **Our sensuality makes our sexuality possible and enjoyable.**

# Patriarchal Religions Fear Female Sensuality

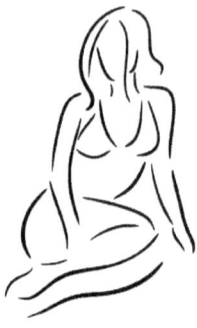

*"Since the dawn of patriarchal religions that put a scolding, punishing father figure God of Wars at the peak of sacredness, dethroning the nurturing mother figure Goddess of Fertility, women's bodies changed in society's eyes from 'sacred powerful birth-giving vessels' to 'bleeding, dirty, disgusting, evil, tempting, and distracting men from their positions of power nasty objects.' Women turned from being the personification of the Goddess to the evil Eve who manipulated Adam to eat the forbidden apple."*
—Sylvia Becker-Hill

The emphasis on modesty, chastity, and covering the body in the five major religions—Christianity, Islam, Hinduism, Buddhism, and Judaism—stems from a combination of psychological drivers—mainly fear, envy, and disgust—cultural norms, and theological beliefs. These religions claim that the underlying psychological drivers include the desire to maintain social order, protect women from objectification, and promote moral and spiritual integrity.

The blind spot in this perspective is not acknowledging the disconnect between humans and nature and their own bodies as part of nature. **The major religions worship the mind over the body as the door to enlightenment or the path to God and believe the body is the seat of all evil, distractions, and sins.**

I believe they are wrong.

I believe all creations—mind and body—are equally as holy or unholy as we choose to see and use them. If there is some kind of divine power/ God/ Goddess/ the Universe/ Nature/ Love/ Life-giving force in the universe… whatever you choose to name "It"—then all creations are divine masterpieces, including the human body.

Yet, don't take my word for it. Do the following beliefs exploring exercise using your own sensuality and interoception and come to your own unique conclusion!

## FLIP - The #1 Acronym for Women's Empowerment

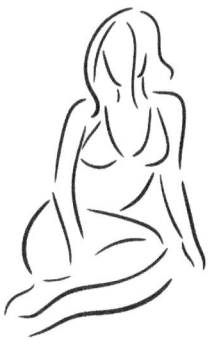

*"An empowered woman is a woman:*
*- who senses her freedom somatically as unquestionable in her body*
*- who loves unconditionally by embodying her inviolable lovability*
*- who authentically shapes her own envisioned identity and*
*- who cares more about her power's positive impact on others*
*than an accumulation of material stuff and status."*
*—Sylvia Becker-Hill*

What does "empowerment" mean? I derived the answers from my clients' results after 27 years of executive coaching, training, and teaching. The most common results my clients share at the end of our projects are:

- They feel freer than ever in their whole life.
- They undoubtedly know they are lovable, experiencing more love in all their relationships, and they learn to love unconditionally using applied neuroscience and attention management.
- They learn tools to shape their own identity and how to show up in the world, growing deliberately into the embodied person they always dreamed of and developing new daily habits.
- They finally have an impact on others and the world that feels utterly satisfying and aligned with their sense of purpose, leaving a legacy.

The acronym FLIP comes from those results: **F**reedom, **L**ove, **I**dentity, **P**ower. I love that the word "flip" also connotes "change," which is my core expertise: change management and applied neuroscience answering the question: "What do we humans need to create lasting positive change?"

Regarding our sensuality and sexuality, I believe we all want to experience more freedom and love, define and curate our own identity, and have the power to create the results and impact we dream of. The first step is to face our painful beliefs that punish us and keep us caged, ashamed, and blocked.

# Getting Punished Through Our Judgemental Thoughts
## - How to FLIP Societal Shoulds Into Sensual Pleasures -

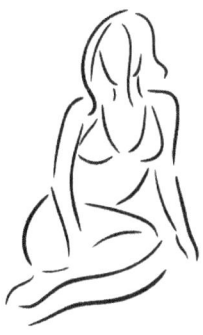

*"Societal conditioning is brutal and insidious.*
*First, someone else imposes judgments.*
*Then we internalize them, and our minds keep blaming us like*
*a broken record, trying to keep us within the safe boundaries of*
*our childhood sphere of societal rules and beliefs."*
—*Sylvia Becker-Hill*

What were the shoulds, rules, or beliefs you grew up with regarding:

- Your body
- Being naked
- Showing skin
- Your sensuality
- Your creativity
- Your beauty
- Your expression
- Your behavior toward the other gender
- Flirting
- Sexual desires, needs, and wants
- Self-pleasuring
- Masturbation

- Sex without being married
- Sex inside a marriage
- Your duties as a woman
- Your freedom as a woman

Here are some examples of beliefs I heard from my clients, friends, or within my own mind over the years:

"A woman's value is defined by her fertility and beauty."

"A woman should be beautiful to look at but not be heard."

"Only ugly women need a good education."

"A woman's body is sinful because it tempts men away from virtue."

"If a woman shows a lot of skin, she is a slut."

"A woman's virginity is her most precious asset."

"When a woman arouses a man, she must accept the consequences."

"All men like to conquer. If you say 'yes' to sex too quickly, you lose the man's respect."

"Dumb women are better in bed than educated, intellectual ones."

"Women in top leadership positions slept their way to the top."

"If you have sex before you're married, you're a slut."

"A woman naturally has fewer sexual partners over her life than a man."

"Sex without emotional attachment is only possible for men."

"Women are addicted to romance and create emotional

entanglement with every man they have sex with."

"Masturbation is unnatural and a sin."

"Without a man, a woman is nothing."

"The most important job for a woman is to find the right husband, ideally by 25. She does that with her beauty and charming personality."

## Journaling Exercise

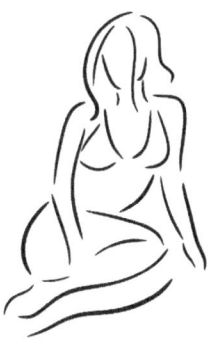

*"The 'truth' of our parents, ancestors, cultures, religions, or whatever collective context… might be a 'truth' we chose to accept as 'true'* **or** *they might turn out upon deeper reflection as intentional lies designed to suppress rebellion against rules* **or** *might turn out to be unproductive beliefs that are outdated.*
**It is our job to distinguish that and choose consciously and wisely.***"*
—*Sylvia Becker-Hill*

Take a pen and write your beliefs in a journal or the margins of this book. Write fast, in your mother language, exactly as you heard them. Set a timer and write for at least 10 minutes.

Now, read those beliefs slowly and **sense in your body** where each belief "sits" and how your body reacts to it.

**Feel**—don't think—the answers to these questions while sensing your body's reactions:

- Does that belief serve your highest well-being?
- Does it feel aligned in your body?
- Is it aligned with how you want to think and feel about your sensuality as a woman?

If the answer to all three questions is yes, great! Keep the belief. If the answer to any of these questions is no, **stay focused** on the sensation inside your body the belief caused and **feel it without resistance**, even if it's uncomfortable. Use curiosity and compassion to stay with the thought until it evaporates somatically from your body and is hard to remember.

This exercise might take a while. Depending on your commitment, you might need several sessions to work through them all. For practical help, use the QR code below for three short videos guiding you through the Emotional Freedom Technique—or "tapping"—to release those beliefs from your body and mind and rewire your brain for new, empowering beliefs.

**After releasing outdated shoulds, it's time to create a list of new sensual freedom-empowering beliefs, pleasure activities, habits, and goals!**

For inspiration, here's my current list:

"I love my body as it is and care for its health and well-being with joy."

"Pleasuring myself is a beautiful expression of my love for myself and my body."

"I move my body daily with full focus for around an hour minimum."

"Health checks, fresh food, natural supplements, good sleep, plenty of water, and grounding rituals are normal for me."

"I find creative ways other than to use food as sensual pleasure."

"I enjoy my sexuality with my husband unabashedly for life."

Your sensuality is why the Divine chose you to experience human life. It allows you to feel both your external and internal world, create pleasure, and expand your consciousness.

**Your sensuality is a perfect, magical, and beautiful divine creation.**

Anyone who claims your sensuality is sinful due to religious reasons, needs suppression due to societal beliefs, or should be left at home due to professional perspectives is mistaken or, worse, misogynistic. They have a distorted view of women, nature, and the spiritual world of consciousness, beauty, and pleasure.

Learning to inhabit your body fully, loving your sensuality, and using it for free expression leads to a creative, pleasure-filled life of beauty and responsible leadership. Someone connected with her sensuality has no desire to harm herself, others, or the environment.

Or as the hippies said: Make love, not war. This applies to your inner life, professional, social, and political realms. **Your sensuality is the door to love and world peace!**

*xoxo,*
*Sylvia*

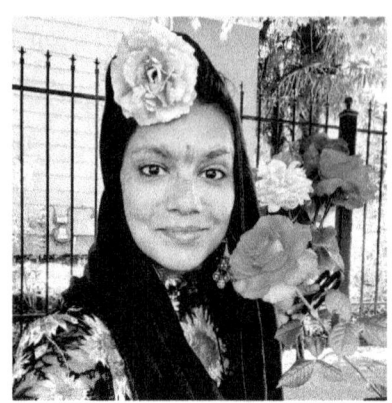

## Aleph Drasmin

Drasmin DreamWorks
Author - Alchemist - Artist

https://www.linkedin.com/in/iamdrasmin/
https://www.facebook.com/drasmindreamworks
https://instagram.com/wordwyrmwomb
https://drasmindreamworks.wixsite.com/addlaw
https://linktr.ee/drasmindreamworks

Tea-sipping earth-worshipping prayerform-dancer and alchemical-poet Drasmin, multiple-published international bestselling author and global platform speaker – meet a neurodivergent visionary dedicated to bridging science, spirit, and love.

Her journey and life inbodies resilience, empowerment, and faith, evident in her temple home, creative works, and nurturing relationships. Within intimate group circles and through daily mindfulness practices, she emphasizes the transformative impact of small daily choices for loving long-term success.

Drasmin integrates eastern and western wisdoms to support Mother Earth's renewal, as well as focuses on language and quantum energetics to harmonize the body's nervous system with all life. Through dream weaving in active sisterhood and in mentorship, she fosters empowerment within her community.

Her magick include a 10 year collection of vision-inspired paintings and spiritual poetry, the CPR deck for mind-heart-body intelligence, multiple solo and co-authored books, and an ever expanding online library of self-guided content empowering thriving in the being human experience.

# Grace Through Fire

By Aleph Drasmin

## 2024

i stood in the kitchen before the sink, in a long see-through black dress, thinking about how to open my chapter in this book, a cool gentle spray of water rinsing the smooshed white berries in my hands. i could feel the male body in the room behind me, watching tv for the first time since i moved in nearly 3 months prior, and the tension between us. two nights ago he had vomited an eviction notice when i dismissed his "obey my rules or else" bark at 11 pm, and even though he asked for a meeting the next day with a mutual friend to mediate, the façade was evident in the days forward.

i stood there, exhausted yet alert, the impending deadline for my first draft looming larger than the eviction notice, wondering how the f$%6 i could write about sensuality when the safety of home no longer existed. i stood there on quicksand for a foundation when it hit me - i was standing in the kitchen in a long see-through black dress with a subtle scent of rosewitchwater spray on my skin, close to a man who no longer made any attempts to hide his displeasure for having me in his home, gently rinsing berries for a light dinner of yogurt, fruit, and nuts… no concern or even thought to the obvious fact a hostile male was a few steps away and could very well and quickly escalate from verbal to physical violence.

only the palpable tension in the room prevented me from laughing out loud! this was it! i was standing in the kitchen fully in my sensual body, anointed with oils and draped under sheer fabric, gently rinsing fruit and preparing a meal that suited the exact needs of my body in that moment. i was dressed for and being me. i had spent the past three hours worshiping my body in an orgasmic meditation, then tending the plants in the garden, a long hot shower followed by my ritual oiling, rolling several herbal cigarettes using a home-made smoking blend, a sunset prayer walk, and now peacefully quietly delicately crafting a nourishing dinner.

yes, the man behind me could fully take advantage of my vulnerability. men are naturally often much stronger physically than women, and the current state of my hands might not allow me to fully defend myself. yet i felt no fear or shame. this realization made me feel gloriously intoxicated.

i had arrived. one breath at a time. i had arrived at this point in my life where i was inbodied (integrated embodiment) in my authentic sovereignty, rooted in my inner peace external circumstances not-withstanding, causally preparing dinner in a sheer black gown that accentuated every curve of my fragrant fabulous figure.

## rewinding time

it was not always like this.

my body through the innocence of childhood was used as a cleansing portal, a human hail-mary to absolve the sins of male doctors-lawyers-pastors-politicians-some seat-of-authority who all shared the belief that the purpose of children, the younger the better, was to pardon their crimes in whatever way they deemed necessary. often these ways were sexual, sometimes with male dogs in heat, as they screamed at the little girls "take that, bitch!" whilst watching and masturbating before spilling their seed into a collective silver chalice that was either forced down the throat of someone, for many years i was "the chosen one", or used in a dark ritual, usually with the blood of a dead child. if any of the seed forced down a child's throat was leaked from the corners of the mouth or spit back out, the child was split in half, crown to tailbone, then hung above the evil altar in the center of the room for 3 days as an example and a warning to anyone who might dare disobey.

this gruesome display of distorted power, however, did not stop some of the children from fighting back. perhaps, their violated bodies in acceptance, they believed they had nothing left to lose and death was preferred over living with the trauma. some others, i believe, genuinely could not take in the entire and sometimes overflowing chalice, gag reflex kicking in. either way, no mercy was ever shown.

as for me, i chose to live – for my little brother whom i was raising as a son. the memory of his eyes and voice kept my eyes free of tears and my throat open for however much they wanted to dump in there. perhaps my stubborn resilience made me a favourite of theirs, and thus i was made to drink of the vile offering more than any of all i saw pass through. i knew for certain i was in their favour when i continued to be dragged back into the room past the age of 11, making me the oldest in the room.

inclusive of sexual perversion was torture, belts and canes to whip, toys and inanimate objects to penetrate, scriptures recited through it all to justify and distort. a part of the evil altar included a human-sized wooden wheel that could be spun on its axis like a roulette wheel, as well as shifted to be either horizontal or vertical. in every ritual, 3 men's names were pulled from a black cauldron marked with gold symbols for the "chosen one" of the day and "the honour of including the altar in today's rites" to do whatever they pleased, all else cackling maniacally as they cheered, drank spirits and smoked, masturbated or had their fun with one or more of the already used children available.

a "sir high priest" in a black hooded cape, as they addressed him, kept order and cauldron. in my nearly 10 years as both witness and unwilling participant, i never saw the same man go twice. once a name was pulled from the black pot, it was filed away in a thick purple cloth bound tome with notes.

the sir never participated, and at the end of the rituals, 3 children were chosen to clean up.

some of the attendees came in masked, and none of the men touched each other. all of them were smart in that no child was ever touched on the face or arms, making it so the bruises that were sure to follow, if the child lived, remained easily hidden. i lost count after 37 how many times i was "the chosen one", sometimes tied face down and unable to witness the horror if the wheel remained horizontal. this was arguably for me the worst of all that occurred, not being able to see who and what was coming.

## breakthrough

a few weeks after turning 15, a golden beacon of hope presented itself.

i had eloped with a man 11 years older than me, together taking an overnight train to a city where we married in his friends' backyard to the music of indian traffic. i was in love, and for the first time since remembrance not thinking of my brother-son whose life had been continuously used as a way to enforce my obedience and silence. my first husband did not know of my sordid past, and, in that moment, in the naivete of youth, believed i was free and that the past has no relevance or importance to and in the present.

it was inching to be the third best day of my life to date, until father broke down the motel room door we were in to find us tangled in each other's arms, still somewhat dressed as we had intended to take our time – the whole day - to consummate our marriage. my dear love was ripped away from me to the screaming broken record of "where's my money, you bastard," fists and steel-toed loafers a whirlwind on a curled form until I jumped onto father's back, yanked his face so I could look straight into his eyes, and screamed, "stop this now or i'm going to tell lucy!" (lucy is my birth mother's name, his wife)

he stopped with a fist mid-air, and i dared not look at the bloody rasping pulp at his feet.

"stop, please." i pleaded softly, still staring into dark orbs mirroring my own, "i will never see him again."

he released the collar tightly held in his left hand and dropped his right fist, then i slid down and quickly gathered my belongings all the while keeping my eyes on the ground. i heard a kick and a grunt, which i perceived to be a final lashing out of father, yet dared not look even as i walked out of the motel room with him right behind, sending a prayer to god-goddess to please let the man live.

i never saw him again, and as the marriage certificate had not yet been delivered to the court house there was nothing to be annulled. 13 years later i learnt he had remarried and fathered 2 children. he lived, blessed be!

on the long train ride back home i did not say a word to father. at first, he glared at me, then as the hours grew without even a tear from my eye, the look turned into brief fear then growing concern. as my own shock abated and i wondered what would happen next, it was this shift in his eyes that gave me both clarity and the golden opportunity. "find a way to get me out of this country asap or mother finds out," i spoke right before we walked into our home to the warm welcome of my excitable mother.

over the days that followed, he fabricated a story, coming home one day with news of a miracle that god had opened an opportunity for me to go to the USA to finish my studies and become a doctor, if i wanted that of course. she danced and screamed in joy across the house while i stood there silent realizing my huge mistake, i had not included my brother-son in the deal, and we both knew it.

my brother was terribly confused at this sudden turn of events and refused to accept i wanted to leave without him. i could not tell him the truth, and he felt it. he did not speak to me until i left a few weeks later, as i knelt before him gifting him my Tintin comic books and asking him to keep them safe for me until i came back for him, a "bye …" without looking at me at the parting gate at the airport in the same city i had been in barely a month prior. it would be the last time i ever saw him.

even though i am a natural-born USA citizen, my mother came with me as i was still underage and could not move to a different country without a legal guardian. as the plane crossed over miles of ocean and land below, the guilt of not being on this journey with my dear brother and son turned into a wall with poisoned soaked coarse spikes that would take nearly 20 years to crumble and neutralize.

## breaking bad

over the years that followed, i was mercifully no longer forced into the room of evil yet the threats for silence remained for nearly a decade. the body, however, had grown addicted to abuse, and the absence of external violence made room for self-inflicted harm. drugs, alcohol, meaningless sex with strangers – nearly 2 years of recklessness until a heroin overdose followed by a forced abortion a few months later shocked me back into human reality. i still had my brother to bring home to me, one way or another.

the self-harm continued, yet i got smart. i learnt how to not mix certain substances and refrain from others, especially needles, and remained unsuspecting as an honours student with a full-time job. i was faithful and loyal to my long-term partners, yet in between had no qualms tossing nameless men and women out of my warm bed at 3 am. i spent countless hours in the gym maintaining a socially accepted physique, and ate relatively healthy and quality food. for creativity, i dabbled in various forms of art and occasionally went on a brief adventure out of town or a longer vacation. i presented a seemingly balanced healthy life, yet as the years rolled on, i grew further disconnected from my body.

## breaking in

over a decade later, i was alcohol and narcotics cold-quit free, and the party hours had been replaced with prayer. i was in my 3rd year of shamanic studies, and the hour I left home on my way to an elder initiation ceremony i began my bleed. i perceived it was just another cycle, stuck a tampon in there, and kept driving. i had never given much thought to my cycle, and this time was no different, even as i continued to spot heavily for the following several weeks. "it's all just part of being a woman."

a few weeks later i went to my first rainbow gathering with a being who had previously attended and invited me weeks after we stopped dating. the 5-hour drive to the forest through cramps and back pain, as well as shooting needle-like pain through my legs, was further aggravated by his incessant complaining about how much i had packed the car. on the way in, we were stopped and roughly searched, which did not silence his tantrum, and we did not arrive at our camp spot and set up till the next rising. by this point, i was losing blood in clots, wracked with pain in every cell, and barely able to hear or see straight when he informed me he had drank all the water i had packed for our 5-day adventure.

to say i was livid is an understatement. i chose silence and walked away. i was brutally ill for the first three days, compounded with poisoning from drinking the contaminated water at the event campgrounds. we barely saw and spoke to each other over the following four days, and when he asked if he could leave without me on the fifth day, i felt ecstatic relief. i had to stay behind for a few more days for the mobile court to roll in, or have a warrant out for my arrest, yet as soon as that was taken care of and i reached cell service nearly 2 hours from the forest, i contacted my naturopath.

a few days later tests confirmed elevated levels of hCG, a hormone that increases during the first few weeks post-conception. there were other markers, i knew the questions to ask because this was not my first miscarriage. plus the combination of my birth doula training, the experience of assisting with several births, pre-med background, and grandmother-mother wisdoms shared over the years.

after receiving this news from the doctor, i took a few weeks to process, both what had happened at the rainbow and how oblivious i had been to what i had been going through for weeks. for all of my meditative practices of presence over the past 3 plus years, i was completely absent from my body.

this was the huge wake-up call to my feminine body. i had allowed others, and myself, to abuse and misuse it for as long as I could remember, conformed to a mold that was not true to my feminine power. it was at this precise moment that i innerstood (lived-experience creates deep inner-understanding) both neglect and self-inflicted harm are abuse. i apologized to my face, breasts, and yoni in front of a mirror, and vowed to my body to become one with my physical temple and especially with my wombspace.

i traced the spiral and discerned the day i began to miscarry was the day i left for the elder initiation, how aligned a total immersion into my higher calling was confirmed and evident in what had followed and now discovered. conception had been with the distasteful man i had recently journeyed with, and, setting my repulsion aside, i meditated deeply on whether to approach him if at all. after three weeks of prayer, i chose to reach out in the hopes at minimum i would have a "spiritual and conscious" friend through the process of grief, this initial mutual thread of attraction shifted post-dating into a brief attempt of friendship.

waking up the day of our plans i felt a horrendous knot in my stomach and throughout the day battled the urge to cancel. i felt proud of myself for putting the ego aside and showing up, for calmly expressing the medical discovery and all relevant evidence, and for briefly expressing some of my emotions around the dynamics of our relationship and his behaviour at the forest gathering. he remained silent throughout my share, which surprised me for he had never shown such restraint during the months we had courted. silence for a few moments, then after a sip of tea from the tiny cup in front of him, we had ordered a pot to share, he looked at me and said, "are you sure it's mine?" i was blown speechless, and it took all of my effort to not hurl the mostly full steaming teapot at him. when dating i had told him i had not been with another man since my last partnership of 7 years had ended nearly a year prior, and we had not had sex for the last 2 years of it. instead, i stood up, murmured a thank you for his time and that i had to go, went home and wept till i fell asleep.

## seasons of time

this was when my relationship with myself as a woman began, delusions ripped off at the denial of this man. was this child his, echoed in my head as i crawled deeper into my womb asking her to show me how to love her and me. i downloaded the clue app and began tracking my cycles, as well as how i felt throughout the days. over the weeks and months that followed, as waves of tears poured out of me for lifetimes and generations of feminine abuse and abandoning, i began to notice a pattern.

somewhere in between the doctor's visit and the turning point, i had begun paying more attention to my body, taking my time to feel the why of exhaustion during undress and her clean suppleness after a shower. growing up in india had me exposed to unrefined coconut oil at a young age, and i had sometimes used it on my skin. after moving to the USA i switched to lotion as that is what everyone else was doing, yet quickly stopped as it always makes my skin cold. after a shower one day, i decided to try the coconut oil again and was pleasantly surprised by how warm and soft my skin felt.

overnight, the extra self-care step of oiling my body straight after a shower became a new practice of meditation. i dedicated to giving my body a slow loving touch every day, and as choices are apt to become after several weeks of consistent repetition, this habit is now a vital and non-negotiable part of my daily self-care as it nourishes all i am so to be and do both personally and professionally.

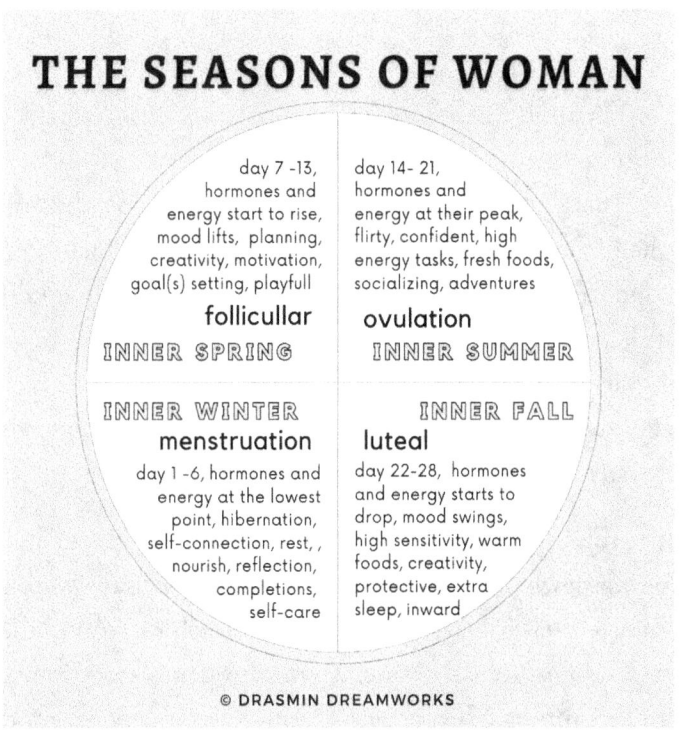

# THE SEASONS OF WOMAN

day 7 -13, hormones and energy start to rise, mood lifts, planning, creativity, motivation, goal(s) setting, playfull

**follicullar**

INNER SPRING

day 14- 21, hormones and energy at their peak, flirty, confident, high energy tasks, fresh foods, socializing, adventures

**ovulation**

INNER SUMMER

INNER WINTER

**menstruation**

day 1 -6, hormones and energy at the lowest point, hibernation, self-connection, rest, , nourish, reflection, completions, self-care

INNER FALL

**luteal**

day 22-28, hormones and energy starts to drop, mood swings, high sensitivity, warm foods, creativity, protective, extra sleep, inward

© DRASMIN DREAMWORKS

years later i realized this was my subtle sensual awaecnian, the simple act of consistent attentive gentle touch to me had cracked open the importance of applying this soft slow way of being into every aspect of life. i went back to research, the voracious student i am, and looked for women empowered with their wombs. through this leap down the rabbit hole, i discovered the seasons of women.

to my delight and surprise, what i learned externally gave voice to the pattern i had already discovered within me over the past few years. i switched from tampons to a reusable menstrual cup, and quit the birth control pills for natural tracking. i grew aware of and learnt how to harness the gift of heightened sensitivity in my body, and continue to grow more familiar with my subtle signals from the innately wise body. eventually, i tapped into the importance of pleasure for life's success, and how to cultivate it daily.

## in the now

with cycle tracking, my eating habits further refined, which had the delicious bonus of saving money! by buying and eating foods according to my seasons, i avoided excess and waste, and was thusly able to acquire the highest quality foods. somewhere along my path, i received my first opportunity to grow a garden, which irrevocably solidified my pleasurefull relationship with food. there is no thing better than harvesting from a garden poured into with sweat-tears-blood and tasting the love. today, growing my own food as much as possible is another vital and non-negotiable way of being.

sometime around my sensual awaecnian, at a tantra retreat, i learnt about boundaries and body-wise consent. the key mind-opening heart-healing soul-empowering revelation was the teaching around the frozen yes - a yes that is actually a no, stemming from tradition, culture, societal programming of expectations, simply not having a good reason to say no, all but a full body yes. over time and with practice, my boundaries grew easier to recognize and stand within, no matter how intimate a relationship. today i continue to deepen in practice to sustain an unshakeable relationship with my mind (meditation), heart (spirituality, aka nature worship), body (food, cycle tracking, and more), and energy (creativity and money), it is easy and preferable to be alone than in the company of those who do not align and support loving sovereign empowered balanced eco-centric way of being.

the cultivation of self, the discovery of sensuality, the application of presence – one breath at a time and one practice at a time strengthening habits and increasing prosperity. i began to apply the seasons of woman to my work life early 2022, and eventually realized i could do more in less time as long as i stayed disciplined and devoted. i continue to schedule life around my seasons, and witness all my interpersonal interactions and passion projects grow in steady harmonic peacefull thriving.

## 3-2-1-4

for today's woman and man, where do you begin?

i could make a list of steps, and refer you to countless other resources.

instead, i pose a question – how badly do you want "it", whatever it is.

everything begins in mind. it is important to check in with why you are choosing to be and do.

for me, "it" was about the promise i had made to me to be healthy so i could be of the highest service to my clients. when i started, being in my sensual power did not register, i felt mostly shame yet refused to let it define or stop me. and now that i have discovered and nurture it daily, i can truthfully say it is the nectar that makes even the most disgusting and annoying tasks both bearable and dare i say fun?!

from shopping for groceries and growing your garden, to preparing your meals and composting or recycling, how you engage with every step, one breath at a time, can be one of pleasure and play.

from paying bills to scrubbing the toilet, from decorating your office to decluttering the attic, from sleep through waking, all presents a choice of attitude to make it easefull and light-hearted, or not.

sensuality is about engaging with pleasure in a non-sexual way…

about seeing the beauty within you and within all around you

about recognizing every breath is a play between life and death

about you being…all that are as you are and choose to be in the now

about you and your every breath weaving with all of life, exisdancsing (to dance in the existence of being) through you and all around you

begINing starts with your gift of free will and your sovereign choice to see it, and choose "it"

# JOIN THE MOVEMENT!
# #BAUW

## Becoming An Unstoppable Woman
## With She Rises Studios

She Rises Studios was founded by Hanna Olivas and Adriana Luna Carlos, the mother-daughter duo, in mid-2020 as they saw a need to help empower women worldwide. They are the podcast hosts of the *She Rises Studios Podcast* and Amazon best-selling authors and motivational speakers who travel the world. Hanna and Adriana are the movement creators of #BAUW - Becoming An Unstoppable Woman: The movement has been created to universally impact women of all ages, at whatever stage of life, to overcome insecurities, and adversities, and develop an unstoppable mindset. She Rises Studios educates, celebrates, and empowers women globally.

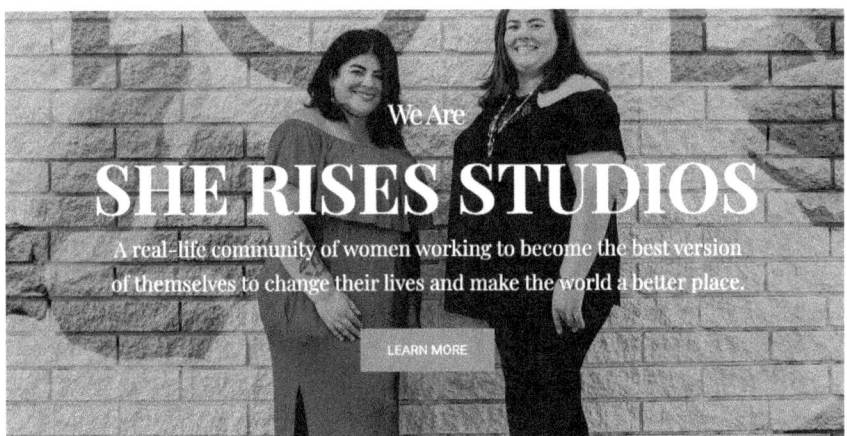

# Looking to Join Us in our Next Anthology or Publish YOUR Own?

She Rises Studios Publishing offers full-service publishing, marketing, book tour, and campaign services. For more information, contact info@sherisesstudios.com

We are always looking for women who want to share their stories and expertise and feature their businesses on our podcasts, in our books, and in our magazines.

## SEE WHAT WE DO

**OUR PODCAST**  **OUR BOOKS**  **OUR SERVICES**

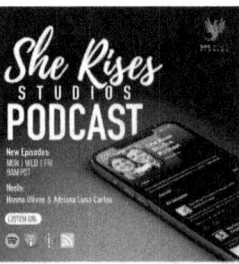
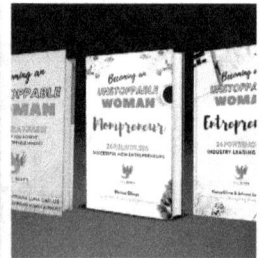
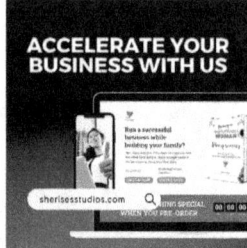

Be featured in the Becoming An Unstoppable Woman magazine, published in 13 countries and sold in all major retailers. Get the visibility you need to LEVEL UP in your business!

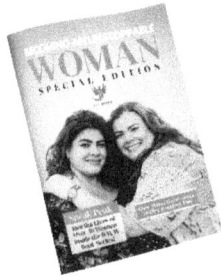 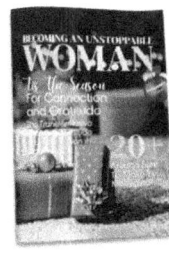 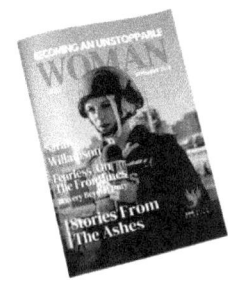

Have your own TV show streamed across major platforms like Roku TV, Amazon Fire Stick, Apple TV and more!

Learn to leverage your expertise. Build your online presence and grow your audience with FENIX TV.
https://fenixtv.sherisesstudios.com/

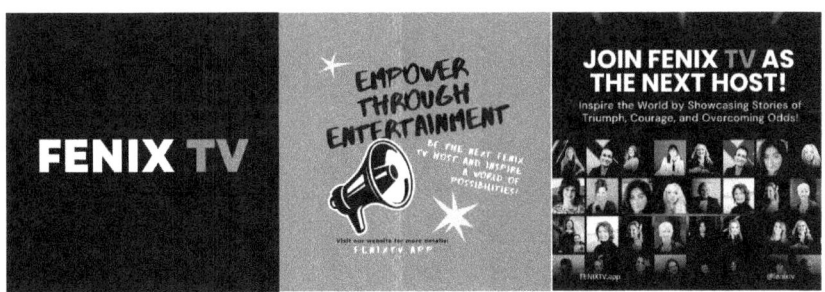

Visit www.SheRisesStudios.com to see how YOU can join the #BAUW movement and help your community to achieve the UNSTOPPABLE mindset.

Have you checked out the *She Rises Studios Podcast?*

Find us on all MAJOR platforms: Spotify, IHeartRadio, Apple Podcasts, Google Podcasts, etc.

**Looking to become a sponsor or build a partnership?**

Email us at info@sherisesstudios.com

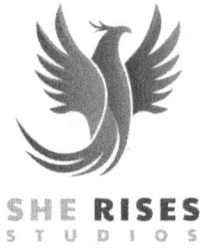

SHE RISES
STUDIOS

www.ingramcontent.com/pod-product-compliance
Lightning Source LLC
Chambersburg PA
CBHW071101120626
46546CB00003B/1244